Obesity:
Its Pathogenesis and Management

Obesity: Its Pathogenesis And Management

Edited by
Trevor Silverstone, DM, MRCP, FRC Psych.

MTP
Medical and Technical Publishing Co Ltd

Published by

MTP
Medical and Technical Publishing Co Ltd
PO Box 55, St Leonard's House,
St Leonardgate,
Lancaster, England

ISBN 0 85200087 1

First published 1975

Type set by Stevenage Printing Limited
Printed by The Garden City Press

Contents

Contributors

David J. Galton, M.D., M. R. C. P.
St Bartholomew's Hospital, London

J. S. Garrow, M.D., PhD., M.R.C.P. Ed.
Medical Research Council, Clinical Research Centre, Harrow, England

Stanislav Hejda, C.Sc.
Institute of Hygiene and Epidemiology, Prague, Czechoslovakia

A. N. Howard, Ph.D.
Department of Investigative Medicine, University of Cambridge

Henry A. Jordan, M.D.
Department of Psychiatry, University of Pennsylvania

Leonard S. Levitz, Ph.D.
Department of Psychiatry, University of Pennsylvania

Kateřina Ošancová, C.Sc.
Institute of Hygiene and Epidemiology, Prague, Czechoslovakia

John P. D. Reckless, M.B., M.R.C.P.(U.K.)
St Bartholomew's Hospital, London

Trevor Silverstone, D.M., M.R.C.P., F.R.C.Psych.
St Bartholomew's Hospital and The German Hospital, London

Orland W. Wooley, Ph.D.
Department of Psychiatry, Medical School, University of Cincinnati

Susan C. Wooley, Ph.D.
Department of Psychiatry, Medical School, University of Cincinnati

Introduction

What I had in mind when I started planning this book was a collection of scholarly essays, each dealing with the problem of obsesity from a particular point of view, which I hoped would be of value to all those working in the field, either as researchers or as therapists. I approached my task in the spirit of an art collector. Such a person must soon recognise that he or she can never, unless possessed of quite extraordinary powers, (and I certainly am not), gather unto himself all the known examples of the works he wishes to collect. Rather he must select, picking out those items which he believes to be most important in the area he is covering. That is what I have tried to do in this book.

As with an art collection, an editor of a series of essays must select both for content and for author. I realise that any such selection is bound to be somewhat arbitrary, but I have tried to include those topics related to obesity which I consider to be, not only the most relevant, but also those in which the most significant theoretical and practical advances are currently being made. The first four of the seven contributions included in the book are concerned with pathogenesis, and the remaining three with management. The first chapter, by Dr. John Garrow, is an overall review of the metabolic influences on body weight as a whole. This is followed by a detailed description, by Drs. Reckless and Galton, of the biochemical pathways involved in adipose tissue metabolism, together with a consideration of how biochemical lesions might lead to increased adiposity and obesity. Epidemiology, a relatively unsung branch of medical science, dealing as it does with large numbers of people rather than with individual patients in the clinic or detailed measurements in the laboratory, has nevertheless made extremely important contributions to our understanding of disease. The review by Drs. Oscancovâ and Hejda of the epidemiological work on obesity provides a sound basis on which further research can develop. The last of the contributions dealing with pathogenesis, that by Drs. Wayne and Susan Wooley, relates to the psychological pressures and attitudes which are brought to bear upon eating behaviour, particularly among obese subjects.

While there is general agreement on the basic therapeutic approach to be adopted in obesity, that is to reduce energy intake to below energy expenditure, there is far less agreement on how best to achieve this aim. The chapters on management present three complementary, rather than alternative approaches. That on dietary treatment by Dr. Alan Howard describes some newer developments in low calorie diets. There follows a critical review by Drs. Jordan and Levitz of the place of behavioural techniques in changing eating behaviour—a relatively novel approach. In the final chapter, I have attempted to place anorectic drugs in perspective, both in terms of our current understanding of appetite and in terms of rational therapy.

I am aware that certain topics related to the problem of obesity have been omitted; to any who feel that the selection has been too idiosyncratic I apologise but do not recant. As I said earlier, the art of collecting is to be selective rather than comprehensive.

The selection of authors is perhaps even more important than that of the contents. Each of the contributors who agreed to participate is an acknowledged authority in his or her discipline and will be familiar to those already working in the field of obesity research. I would like to take this opportunity of thanking them all most sincerely for being not only wise and industrious (after all I chose them for that) but for also being so helpful and understanding.

I hope this collection of scientific essays lives up to the hopes I had for it when I started—it certainly afforded me a good deal of pleasure in the making.

Trevor Silverstone

1

The Regulation of Body Weight

J. S. Garrow

The regulation of body weight has been most intensively studied in the laboratory rat. If it is given unlimited access to a standard laboratory chow the rat grows along a predictable curve: normally it is weaned at about three weeks of age, when it weighs perhaps 20 g; for the next five weeks growth is rapid, then the rate of increase slackens. Similar growth curves for the human infant are familiar to paediatricians: normal birthweight is about 3.5 kg, and growth is then rapid to reach about 10 kg at one year, and subsequently the curve flattens until the adolescent growth spurt is reached. Children of lower than average birthweight tend to grow in parallel with the average weight curve, so in general small babies remain smaller than average, and large ones tend to remain relatively large. Similar 'programming' of the growth curve is easily demonstrated in rats, but if a rat is prevented from following its normal growth channel, for example by undernutrition, the long-term effect depends on the exact stage of development at which the nutritional deprivation occurred. McCance has reviewed the interactions of food, growth and time in the development of many species. For example if baby rats are suckled 15 to a mother, and are then fed *ad libitum* they will never catch up with littermates who were suckled three to a mother and thereafter allowed access to exactly the same diet. On the other hand if at the age of nine weeks normal rats are held back in growth by undernutrition they will rapidly make good this lost growth as soon as they have unlimited food again. If undernutrition is prolonged it becomes evident that different tissues within the same animal are differently affected. The chronically undernourished piglet will grow very slowly, but the development of the teeth is set back less than that of the jaws by shortage of food, so the molars become impacted because there is no room for them to erupt normally.

All this suggests that animals, and even tissues, have a 'normal' growth pattern to which they will conform unless prevented from doing so by nutritional constraints, and that the effects of these constraints will vary according to the period of development at which they are applied. This concept is of some importance when we come to consider the pathogenesis and management of human obesity. In the obese human body, weight clearly has not been adequately regulated, or possibly it has been regulated in relation to a misplaced set point. This interpretation may lead to the fatalistic view expressed by Astwood[2] 'I wish to propose that obesity is an inherited disorder and due to a genetically determined defect in an enzyme: in other words that people who are fat are born fat, and nothing much can be done about it'. If it is really true that obesity is an incurable disease, then we might as well accept the fact, and stop tormenting obese patients by applying futile dietary restrictions. There are several authorities who conclude that the dietary treatment of obesity is virtually hopeless[3] and hence that 'One might well question whether refractory obese patients should be treated at all'[4].

However, before we all join in this chorus of despair, it is very important to establish that the pessimism is justified, otherwise the prophesy of therapeutic failure is sure to be a self-fulfilling one. All too often the obese patient comes to the doctor convinced that his or her case is beyond mortal help, and if the doctor readily agrees the chances of success are vanishingly small. Personally I believe that these jeremiads about the impossibility of treating obesity are unjustified, and do a great disservice to both doctors and their obese patients. Certainly obesity is difficult to treat, and the best you may be able to hope for is an improvement in fitness, appearance and morale in the patient, rather than a return to the normal range in weight, and these modest objectives may be attainable only after many months of effort by both the patient and the doctor. However the same could equally truthfully be said of much of medical care: in the management of strokes, coronary thrombosis, osteoarthritis, drug addiction and many forms of mental disease the 'cure' rate (in the sense of complete return to normal function) is at least as low as it is in obesity, yet so far as I know it has not been suggested that these conditions are not worth treating.

In this chapter an attempt will first be made to clarify the relationship between body weight and obesity. The gloom which pervades 'refractory' obese patients is often based on the observation that despite keeping to a reducing diet they did not lose weight. At first sight this is indeed evidence that diet cannot cure their particular type of obesity, but a better understanding of the possible short-term variations in body composition may help them to accept that an increase in body weight (temporarily) is not incompatible with a decrease in energy stores, and hence in the long term diet will be effective in reducing body weight. Next the mechanisms will be reviewed by which body weight and energy balance are normally maintained in animals and man, and some observations will be made about the way in which these control mechanisms may be influenced. Finally an attempt will be made to assess the extent to which, in man, obesity is 'an inherited disorder . . . and nothing much can be done about it'[2].

THE RELATIONSHIP OF BODY WEIGHT TO OBESITY

Obesity is a state in which an excess of fat accumulates[5]. To put this definition to practical use it is necessary to determine, in a given individual, how much fat he contains, and then to decide if this is 'an excess': neither of these tasks is easy. Methods by which the amount of fat, and other body constituents, can be estimated will be discussed in some detail later, but the criterion of 'excess' fat can be dealt with here.

Life insurance companies are interested in the life expectancy of candidates for insurance, and in particular they are concerned to identify those people in whom life expectancy is shorter than average, since obviously if such people are insured at normal premiums the company will be liable to make very little profit from the transaction. Of the various factors which have been shown to diminish life expectancy, obesity is among the most important, and for want of any better criterion of obesity standards of weight-for-height have been calculated. The underwriter is not concerned with individual cases: he wants a general rule which will enable him to calculate the appropriate premium for any candidate for insurance[6], so there are tables of 'desirable weight' for men and women of different heights. These tables distinguish between 'small, medium and large frame' individuals, but it is not clear how the frame size appropriate to a given person should be established.

Obesity defined by relative weight (that is, weight compared with desirable weight for height) is not necessarily a state in which there is excess fat, and conversely it is possible to have almost as much fat as lean tissue but still be in the desirable weight-for-height range[7]. The fallibility of relative weight as a criterion of obesity was dramatically shown when, in 1942, the United States Navy rejected as unfit some extremely muscular football players, since their weight for height exceeded the desirable range[8]. The opposite error, of passing as normal individuals who have very large fat burdens, but little lean tissue, so they appear in the desirable range of weight for height, is most likely to occur in women over sixty years[7]. Despite these theoretical disadvantages of using relative weight as a criterion of obesity, for most purposes it is the best, and certainly the most convenient, measurement. It is on the basis of relative weight that life insurance actuaries have shown increased mortality associated with overweight, and in the Framingham study[9] overweight is the most powerful single determinant of cardiovascular disease. Other complications of obesity, such as osteoarthritis of weight-bearing joints, are presumably related to the actual load on these joints, rather than to the proportion of fat in the body. Perhaps the most compelling of all arguments for the use of weight as a measure of obesity is that it can be easily and accurately measured, so that progress in the treatment of obesity can be followed by weight loss, at least in the long term. The significance of short-term fluctuations in body weight is discussed below.

Lean body mass and adipose tissue

The excessive amount of fat in an obese patient is stored in adipose tissue. This is situated mainly in the subcutaneous layer, but there are also deep sites which contain adipose tissue, particularly in the mesentery of the gut, around the kidneys, and (conveniently in the rat) as a pad next to the epididymis. The remainder of the tissues of the body, other than the adipose tissue, is the lean body mass. Analyses of the chemical composition of human adipose tissue have been reviewed in some detail elsewhere[10] and are discussed more fully in Chapter 2: on average in normal subjects adipose tissue is about 78% fat, 18% water and 3% protein, but in obese subjects the amount of fat increases relative to the cytoplasm of the fat cell, so the chemical analysis shows about 83% fat, 14% water and 2% protein.

Our knowledge of the chemical composition of the lean body mass is based chiefly on the analysis of six adult cadavers[11–14]. The amount of fat in these bodies varied from 4.3 to 27.9%, and when the fat was removed the amount of water, protein and potassium in the fat-free body is shown in Table 1.1. On average these fat-free bodies contained 72.5% water, 20.5% protein, and the remaining 7% is mostly mineral (largely in bone), glycogen, and substances such as nucleic acids. In Table 1.1 the amount of potassium in the fat-free bodies is shown: on average, in the four bodies in which this measurement was made, the concentration is 69 mmol K kg^{-1} fat-free weight. All the bodies were those of men except the one aged forty-two years: this was a woman who committed suicide

TABLE 1.1 *The contribution of water and protein to the fat-free weight of six adult bodies*
(for sources of these data see text)

Age (yrs)	Water ($g\ kg^{-1}$)	Protein ($g\ kg^{-1}$)	Remainder ($g\ kg^{-1}$)	Potassium ($mmol\ kg^{-1}$)	K:N ratio ($mmol\ g^{-1}$)
25	728	192	77	71.5	2.29
35	775	165	60	—	—
42	733	192	75	73.0	2.38
46	674	234	92	66.5	1.78
48	730	206	64	—	—
60	704	238	58	66.6	1.75
Mean	725	205	71	69.0	2.05

by drowning. There is some evidence that the potassium content of the lean body mass in women is less than that in men[15], but in this case the potassium concentration of 73 mmol kg^{-1} is higher than that of any of the male bodies.

Measurement of the proportion of lean and adipose tissue in living subjects

It was noted above that if we are to put to practical use the definition of obesity as 'a state in which excessive fat accumulates' we must be able to measure the amount of fat in a living subject. There are several ways in which this can be done, but none is very convenient and reliable. The most reliable methods are least convenient, and vice versa. A fuller account of these techniques is given elsewhere[10].

Fat-soluble gas methods

If the subject breathes an atmosphere containing a known concentration of a fat-soluble gas, such as krypton or cyclopropane, this gas will dissolve in his body fat until an equilibrium is reached in which the partial pressure of gas in the fat equals the partial pressure in the inspired air. At that stage no further uptake of fat-soluble gas will occur. The solubility of these gases in fat at body temperature is accurately known, so if the equilibrium concentration and the amount of gas taken up is measured the total body fat can be calculated. This method of estimation is theoretically excellent, and in practice very reproducible estimates of body fat have been obtained in human subjects with either krypton[16] or cyclopropane[7]. The disadvantage of the technique is that it involves sealing the subject into an airtight breathing circuit for the time needed to reach equilibrium, which is a matter of hours.

Calculation of lean body mass from total body potassium

The data in Table 1.1 show that the potassium content of the fat-free body is fairly constant at about 69 mmol kg^{-1}. It is fortunate for students of human body composition that potassium has a naturally occurring isotope, ^{40}K, which emits gamma rays of a characteristic and high energy (1.46 mEv), and has a radioactive half-life which is long relative to the human lifespan. In effect this means that each gramme of potassium, whether in the human body or not, sends out about three of these gamma rays per second, and since they are of high energy there is a good chance that, wherever in the body they may originate and whatever direction they travel, they will eventually emerge from the skin. If suitable apparatus is used these gamma rays (or a representative sample of them) can be detected and counted, and hence the total potassium content of the body can be calculated. Since the potassium in the body is almost exclusively in the lean component the lean body mass can be calculated, and if this is subtracted from total body weight, adipose tissue mass is estimated.

For the subject this method of determining body fat is more convenient than the fat soluble gas method, since it is only necessary to lie or sit in a gamma spectrometer for 10-30 minutes (depending on the design of the spectrometer) for a measurement of total body potassium to be made. However the theoretical difficulties of this method are considerable. It is true that the average potassium concentration in the lean body mass is about 69 mmol kg^{-1}, but the individual tissues which make up the lean body have very different potassium concentrations: for example skin 23.7, kidneys 57.0, heart 66.5, liver 75.0, brain 84.6 and muscle 92.2 mmol kg^{-1} respectively[17,18]. The constancy of the average lean body therefore depends on the proportions in which these tissues are represented also fairly constant. In well nourished adults it is reasonable to assume that these tissues are represented in fairly constant proportions, but in extreme cases of nutritional disturbance, such as severe infantile malnutrition, the ratio of brain, skin and bone may be greatly increased relative to muscle, and hence it is difficult to make a true estimate of lean body mass from total body potassium.

Methods based on total body water

The fat-free body contains about 72.5% water (see Table 1.1). It is fairly easy to measure total body water, by giving a known dose of isotopically labelled water (deuterium or tritium oxide), and determining the dilution of this water in body fluids after equilibrium has been attained. If, for example, 10 g of labelled water is given, and after about 4 hours the concentration of labelled water in blood is 1:5000, it follows that the volume in which the tracer was distributed was 50 kg water. If the assumption is made that this is the water in the fat-free body, then the fat-free mass is 50/0.725 kg, or 69 kg. If the total body weight of the subject is 80 kg it follows that total body fat is 11 kg.

This technique for measuring body fat is widely used, and for subjects who are not too obese it is probably the best compromise between convenience and accuracy. Unfortunately in very obese subjects the method becomes unreliable. It is assumed that lean body mass contains 72.5% water, and that all the water is in the lean body mass: in very obese subjects neither assumption is necessarily valid. Consider a patient with 100 kg of adipose tissue: this tissue will contain about 14 kg of water and 2 kg protein. It may be argued that this water and protein should be considered part of the lean body mass, since it related to the cytoplasm of the adipose cell, but if this is done the fundamental assumption that the water content of the lean body mass is 72.5% cannot be upheld, since the water content of fat-free adipose tissue is about 87%. The other major problem in estimating fat-free weight from total body water in very obese subjects is that these subjects often have an excessive amount of extracellular fluid, which may be clinically evident as edema. Clearly, edema fluid will be included in a measurement of total body water, and will therefore give a falsely high estimate of lean body mass, and hence a falsely low estimate of total body fat.

Methods based on body density

The density of human fat at body temperature is 0.900, mineral is 3.00, protein about 1.34 and water 1.00. Obviously it is impossible to calculate the proportions of these four variables from mean body density, but if the assumption is made that the mixture of water, protein and minerals which makes up the fat-free body has an average density of 1.10, then it is possible from a measurement of whole body density to assign a ratio of fat to fat-free body. To measure body density it is necessary to measure the weight and volume of the body: measurement of weight is easy, but volume is difficult. Various techniques have been tried, but the most commonly used is to weigh the subject first in air and then submerged in water. The apparent loss in weight when under water equals the weight of water displaced, as Archimedes pointed out, and from this the volume immersed can be calculated.

The disadvantages of the underwater weighing method are that it is troublesome and even alarming to some subjects, and the volume immersed is not the same as the volume of the body tissues: obviously gas in the lungs and in the gut will also contribute to the volume of water displaced when the subject is totally immersed. It is possible to measure, and correct for, the gas in the lungs, but intestinal gas is more difficult to measure. Recently a modification of the water displacement method has been developed[19]. The subject is almost completely submerged in water in a vertical tank, the tank is sealed for a short time and a known volume of water is withdrawn. The amount of water in the tank is known, and the pressure drop when some is withdrawn is measured. From these data it is possible to obtain an accurate estimate of both the volume of water and also the volume of air in the tank at the moment when it was sealed, since air in the subject's lungs and gut, as well as that surrounding his head, will expand when the pressure is reduced. It may be that this will prove to be the most accurate of all methods for measuring changes in fat content in a human subject. It shares with underwater weighing the problem of accurately defining the density of the fat-free body, and hence it will probably not be as reliable a method for estimating the total amount of fat as the fat-soluble gas method.

Measurements of subcutaneous fat thickness

Since the largest depots of adipose tissue are subcutaneous, an estimate of the amount of subcutaneous fat gives a good index of obesity. This is most conveniently done by pinching up a fold of skin, with the underlying fat layer, and measuring the thickness of this fold with suitably designed calipers[20]. Sites at which it is fairly easy to obtain a skinfold in normal subjects are over the triceps muscle, at the lower angle of the scapula, and just above the iliac crest. Regression equations have been derived relating the thickness of skinfolds at these and other sites to the total fat content determined by other methods, such as underwater weighing.

The limitations of the skinfold caliper method are that only a few sites are sampled, and in very obese subjects it is often impossible to obtain a valid skinfold measurement at any site, since there is not enough loose skin on the limbs to make a fold, while the folds which appear spontaneously on the trunk are too large to measure with the caliper. The second difficulty can be overcome by using ultrasonic apparatus, by which the depth of the fat layer can be calculated from the time taken for a pulse of ultrasound to travel from the skin to the underlying muscle and return[21]. The problem of sampling is more difficult to overcome. People differ in fat distribution[22], and although in theory it might be possible to correct for these differences by somatotype photography, in practice it would be a very tedious calculation. Soft-tissue radiography has also been used to measure subcutaneous fat thickness, but the problem of sampling remains.

RELATIONSHIP OF CHANGE IN BODY WEIGHT TO ENERGY BALANCE

From the discussion above it will be evident that relative body weight is a fairly good index of obesity, but in those subjects in whom it is likely to be misleading (such as athletes and elderly women) there are other methods by which the amount of adipose tissue can be measured. Unfortunately none of these methods is very accurate, so we cannot say with certainty that a patient who has lost, say, 500 g in weight has lost fat or lean tissue, or even water. In terms of energy balance the distinction is important, since 500 g fat has an energy value of 4500 kcal, an equal weight of lean body mass about 450 kcal, and water has no energy value.

Obese patients need to lose fat, not merely weight. To lose fat it is necessary to create a negative energy balance, so the energy content of the fat is used to make up the deficit between energy intake and expenditure. Producing and sustaining a negative energy balance is difficult and tedious, so obese patients are all too easily induced to adopt apparently easy routes to weight loss. Notorious among these is the use of diuretics, which cause a temporary decrease in body water (and hence body weight) without in any way affecting energy balance. The obese patient thus treated is worse off than before: she has observed in herself a rapid, effortless, and apparently beneficial weight loss under the influence of some pills, and naturally hopes for similar success again. Obviously this hope cannot be fulfilled without the use of even more powerful diuretics which would eventually lead to a dangerous state of dehydration. Thus the patient has gained nothing useful, and has probably become even less able to accept the slow steady weight loss produced by a negative energy balance which is the only eventual road to her salvation.

Even with a reducing diet weight loss does not always occur, and it is necesary to offer an explanation for this, or the patient will become disenchanted with dieting also. The extent of weight loss depends on the energy value of the component of the body which is being lost. For the purpose of this discussion it is necessary to consider only three components of body weight which are illustrated in Figures 1.1 and 1.2. Mineral has no energy value, and changes little in weight in healthy subjects, so it will not be considered further.

Figure 1.1 is a schematic representation of a normal adult male weighing 69 kg. The components relevant to energy balance are the lean body mass, adipose tissue, and glycogen/water pool. In round numbers the lean body mass may be considered to be a mixture of 10 kg protein and 40 kg water, making 50 kg in all. Adipose tissue can be represented by 10 kg fat and 5 kg water, a total of 15 kg. The glycogen/water pool is shown in the diagram as a collapsible bellows: the total weight of this compartment is 4 kg, and it is made up of 800 g glycogen and 3200 g of water.

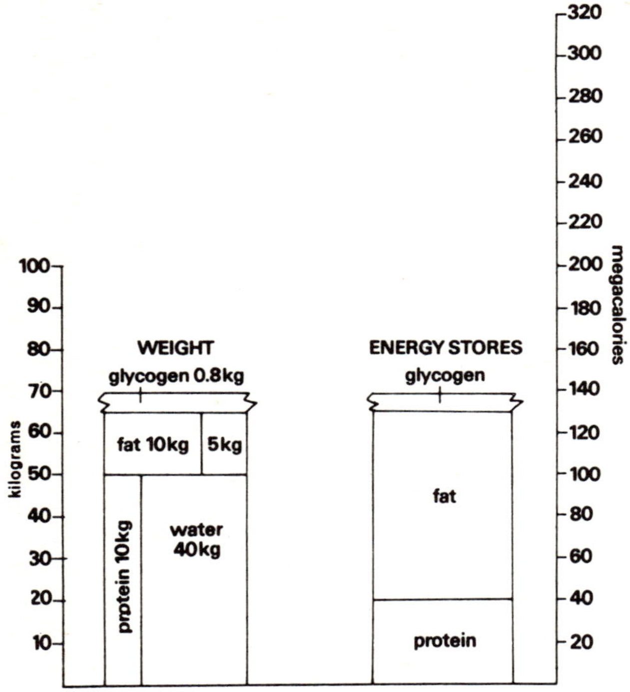

FIGURE 1.1 Body weight and energy stores of a normal adult weighing about 69 kg (11 stones)

The energy value of protein and glycogen is 4 kcal g^{-1}, and of fat 9 kcal g^{-1}. Thus in this simplified model the body of a normal adult consists of three components: the lean body mass and the glycogen/water pool each have an energy value of 0.8 kcal g^{-1} (since in each case the protein or glycogen is associated with four times its weight of water), and the adipose tissue has an energy value of 6 kcal g^{-1}, since the fat is associated with half its weight of water. It is obvious from this simple model that if the subject is in negative energy balance to the extent of 1000 kcal, and this is met entirely at the expense of either the lean body mass or the glycogen pool, the decrease in body weight will be about 1250 g, while if the energy deficit is met entirely from adipose tissue the decrease in body weight will be about 167 g, since the energy value of adipose tissue is about 7.5 times greater than that of the other components.

Figure 1.2 indicates in a similar way the approximate body composition of an adult man who has become obese, and who has now reached 99 kg. In this diagram the lean body mass and glycogen pool have been assumed to remain constant and the obesity is attributed

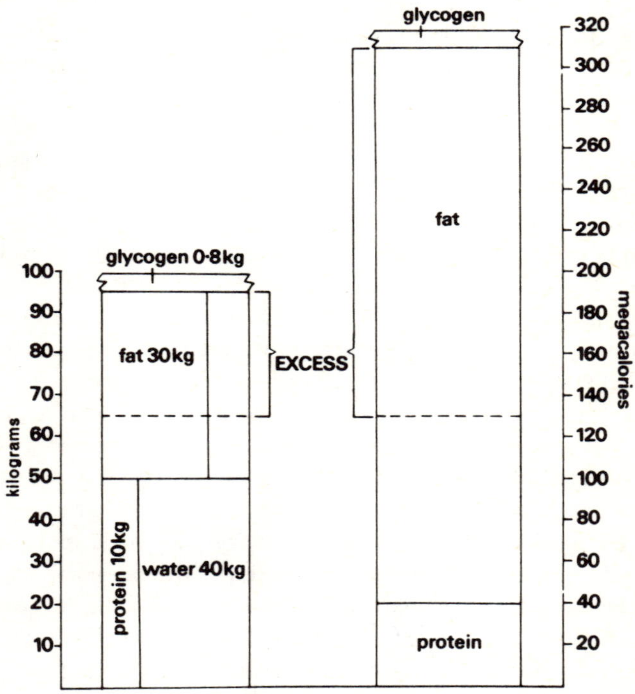

FIGURE 1.2 Obese adult weighing 99 kg (15 stones). Excess fat would supply total energy for three months.

entirely to an increase of 30 kg in the adipose tissue. In fact the situation is not quite so simple as this, and there will be changes in other body components which are discussed more fully elsewhere[10] but the model is substantially accurate. The important point which is shown in Figure 1.2 is that although the increase in body weight of the obese subject is not very great the increase in energy stores is huge, since an extra 30 kg of adipose tissue contains 20 kg of fat, and this is equivalent to 180 000 kcal, or more than the total energy stores of the lean subject.

We may now return to the problem of the obese patient who does not lose weight despite keeping to a reducing diet. There are three possible explanations for this phenomenon, which will be considered in order of probability.

The most likely, but by no means the only, reason for 'refractory' obesity is that the patient has not in fact kept to a diet as low in energy as was intended. This is not necessarily due to deliberate cheating: there may be genuine misunderstandings about the rules of dieting. This aspect of the treatment of obesity is considered further in Chapter 5.

The next most probable explanation for failure to lose weight, even when a correctly designed reducing diet is scrupulously followed, is an alteration of the proportions of the body components shown in Figures 1.1 and 1.2. Obviously this effect can only explain temporary failure to lose weight, since there is a limit to the extent to which body composition can change. However the effect is an important one, since if it is not understood it may destroy the morale of the patient. Usually the complaint is either 'I lose weight quite well when I start on a diet, but after about a week I hardly lose anything', or alternatively 'I have to absolutely starve myself to lose weight, and if I take even a slice or two of bread my weight increases, even though I am still keeping far below the calorie level permitted on the diet'. Both these complaints may be quite true, and are not difficult to explain. The patient who starts on a reducing diet and is, say, 500 kcal per day in negative energy balance will at first supply this energy deficit from the glycogen/water pool, and hence may obtain a weight loss of about 600 g/day. After about a week the glycogen pool is exhausted, so the energy deficit is met mainly by adipose tissue, so the rate of weight loss for 500 kcal-worth of adipose tissue is only about 80 g per day. Since the average bathroom scales have an error of some 400 g from day to day, or even between repeat weighings on the same day, it is not difficult to understand that a patient who had observed a rate of weight loss of 600 g/day for the first week should regard this as 'losing weight quite well' and when the inevitable decrease to the barely detectable rate of 80 g/day, she will conclude that she 'hardly loses anything'. If at this stage she is so disheartened that she gives up the diet her weight will rapidly increase as the glycogen stores are refilled, and hence all her worse fears about the inefficacy of dieting are confirmed.

The alternative complaint that following virtual starvation weight increases with a slice or two of bread can also be explained on the basis of the effects of starvation and carbohydrate intake on sodium balance. It has been known for many years that after starvation, a small amount of carbohydrate would inhibit sodium excretion, and hence cause an increase in body water and body weight. It is unlikely that the mechanism of this effect is the same as that described above, since the amount of carbohydrate required to produce the effect is very small, and it is difficult to imagine that the retention of sodium was associated with an increase in the storage of glycogen in a subject who is still in strongly negative energy balance. Studies have been made of the electrolyte balance of subjects who were fed a very small amount of carbohydrate for six days, then starved for seven days, and finally re-fed the same small amount of carbohydrate for another six days[23]. Although the total energy intake during the last period was only 610 kcal/day, and the subjects were certainly in negative energy balance, body weight significantly increased. The authors were able to show that the ketoacidosis of starvation provides the necessary ions for the excretion of sodium, but that when a small amount of carbohydrate is given, sufficient to stop the ketosis and rapid protein breakdown, there is a temporary sodium retention which accounts for the weight gain.

A simple practical way to discover if a given patient really does maintain weight on a diet providing 800-1200 kcal/day, is to persuade the patient to try taking either two or three pints of milk a day, and nothing else except water and acaloric flavouring such as tea or coffee. This diet, though dull, has the merit of being of accurately known energy content, since milk provides about 400 kcal/pint. It is readily available, and easily measured out, and contains a low and constant amount of both sodium and carbohydrate. It is not suitable as a long term diet, except in unusual circumstances, since it is deficient in iron and vitamins, but as a test diet for a week or two it is useful, and certainly no obese patient will come to any nutritional harm by restricting themselves to two pints of milk per day, plus water as required, for a week or two.

The least likely explanation for a patient to fail to lose weight on a properly designed, and accurately observed, reducing diet is that they have so reduced their metabolic rate that they can maintain energy balance on a very small energy intake. This is the explanation which most 'refractory' obese patients favour as the cause of their difficulties, but on careful investigation the two previous explanations are found to be more commonly correct.

THE CONTROL OF ENERGY BALANCE IN MAN

Unlike the laboratory rat, man does not accurately balance his daily energy intake against daily energy expenditure. It is obvious that in the long term, if body weight is to be maintained at a fairly constant level, there must be a balance between the intake and expenditure of energy, and Edholm and his colleagues have conducted exhaustive experiments to elucidate the manner in which the control system operates, but the answer is extraordinarily elusive.

Figure 1.3 is taken from a study by Edholm *et al.*[24] They measured the total energy intake and expenditure of twelve military cadets over a period of fourteen days. In Figure 1.3 the daily energy intake of each cadet is plotted against the expenditure the same day. The range of

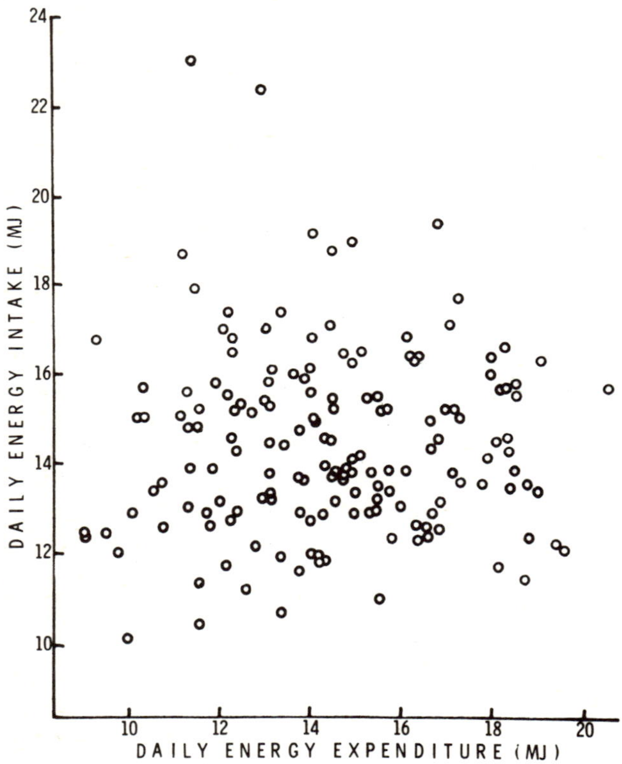

FIGURE 1.3 Relationship between daily energy intake and daily energy expenditure of twelve military cadets over a period of fourteen days. From Edholm *et al.*[24]

intake and expenditure within a group of fit young men, undergoing the same course of military training, is remarkable, and so is the total lack of correlation in daily intake and expenditure for each individual. Analysis of these and other data have shown that the results illustrated in Figure 1.3 are not simply the result of a time lag in response: that is, intake does not correlate with the previous day's expenditure, nor that of two days previously. In this study the average intake of all the cadets for 14 days was 3432 kcal/day, and the average expenditure was 3416 kcal/day. This has been quoted as evidence that, although energy balance is not maintained from day to day, it is accurately maintained over a period of two weeks. This is not a valid interpretation of Edholm's results. If the mean energy intake for each cadet is plotted against the mean energy expenditure of the same cadet for the two-week period, there is no close match in ten of the twelve subjects. Only two cadets managed to maintain balance within 150 kcal/day, and in the remainder the imbalance ranged up to 800 kcal/day for the fortnight, making a total error of over 11 000 kcals. By statistical testing there is no evidence of a significant correlation between intake and expenditure in these cadets: the correlation coefficient is only 0.10.

It is not practicable to make accurate measurements of food intake and the nature and duration of every activity of subjects for more than a period of two weeks: even this length of study put a considerable strain on the stamina of both subjects and investigators. In view of the large errors in energy balance which have been shown in the studies of Edholm and others, it is reasonable to examine the evidence that there is accurate control of body weight in normal people, and hence that obese patients have a defect in their control mechanism. There is a danger of being trapped in a circular argument: if we start with the proposition that normally body weight is controlled at a constant value, we will inevitably conclude that individuals in whom body weight is not constant are not normal individuals. To avoid this trap it is necessary to abandon preconceptions about what constitutes normality, and observe the magnitude of changes in body weight which occur in the population as a whole.

The stability of body weight in the general population

It is obviously fruitless to consider changes in body weight in a sample of the population who are trying to change their body weight: for example obese patients under treatment. The problem is to find a representative sample of the population who are regulary and accurately weighed, but who are not particularly concerned to influence their weight in any particular direction. The best source of such data is probably from the Framingham Heart Disease study. This was started in 1948 in the town of Framingham, near Boston, and involves 5209 adults who were between thirty and fifty-nine years of age at that time. Every two years since enrollment in the study, these subjects have been given a thorough physical examination which was aimed mainly at detecting cardio-vascular disease, but which included accurate measurement of body weight. Gordon and Kannel[9] have recently reported the results of the first eighteen years, covering ten examinations. The fluctuations in body weight which were found in the 1277 men and 1690 women who completed all ten examinations are shown in Figure 1.4. The original measurements were reported in lb and the figure is divided in kg, hence the columns do not exactly fit the graduations.

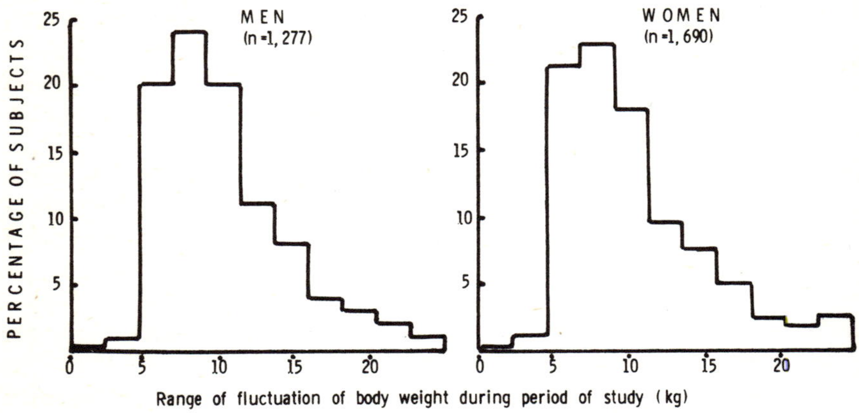

FIGURE 1.4 Fluctuations in body weight during eighteen years in Framingham study. Age at entry thirty to fifty-nine years.

It is evidently very rare for an individual to maintain constant weight within 5 kg over eighteen years, the average range of fluctuation is 10 kg, and about 18% show fluctuations of more than 15 kg. The authors comment: 'While average differences between highest and lowest weights for individuals are large (over 21 lb), this chiefly reflects short-term fluctuation. Persistent changes occur very slowly, and weight at one age is closely related to weight in later life for most people.' Other studies have also shown that, whatever the mechanism may be which keeps body weight fairly constant during adult life, this control system tolerates departures of some 10 kg from the 'set point' weight in most people[10] (see also Chapter 3). To conclude this discussion of the control of body weight, and its relationship to obesity, three more questions must be considered:

First, what is the nature of the control system which normally regulates body weight in man?

Second, is obesity a result of the failure of this mechanism, or is it that the 'set point' to which the mechanism regulates has for some reason been set too high?

Third (since no very confident answer can be given to either of the first two questions), what, in our present state of knowledge, should we try to do in order to cure or prevent obesity?

The nature of the control mechanism regulating body weight

The long-term regulation of body weight is essentially a problem of energy balance. In the short term, as explained above, change in body weight does not necessarily follow changes in the body energy stores, but over a period of years, or where large changes in body weight are involved (such as 10 kg), inevitably errors in energy balance are involved. In experimental animals it has been shown that energy balance is maintained by control of energy intake, and three main theories have been put forward to explain how the state of energy balance is sensed in order to inform the centres controlling feeding behaviour. These theories will not be discussed in detail, since full accounts can be read in the reviews quoted below, and also because it is evident that none of these theories, nor any combination of them, can adequately explain the regulation of body weight in man.

The glucostatic theory, and its relation to other theories has been reviewed by Mayer[25]. Briefly the hypothesis is that the change in glucose concentration in the blood perfusing the nuclei in the hypothalamus is the signal which initiates the drive to eat or to stop eating. The main problem about this theory is that blood glucose is so labile that it is difficult to imagine a long-term regulation based on so transient a signal, and experimental manipulation of the blood sugar (for example by injection of glucose or insulin) does not always give results consonant with this theory. However, it is undeniable that hypoglycaemia is one of the factors causing a drive to eat, so the glucostatic theory cannot be completely invalid. The thermostatic theory has been reviewed by Brobeck[26,27]: this postulates that the increase in body temperature which follows a meal, and which results from accelerated metabolism, is the signal to which the hypothalamus is sensitive. Again the theory is only partially satisfactory, but animals kept in a cold environment will greatly increase their food intake in order to maintain normal body temperature, so cold is another source of the drive to eat. The weakness of both the above theories is that it is difficult to understand how either can account for the ability of rats to correct for very large and prolonged deviations from energy balance. For example Cohn and Joseph[28] fed rats double the normal rations by gavage for a period of three months, at which stage they had attained a body weight of 500-600 g, while control littermates were only 300-350 g. Both groups of rats were then allowed unlimited access to the same pelleted diet, and the overfed animals spontaneously ceased to eat, or ate only sparingly, for two to three weeks, and after thirty to forty days the two groups of rats attained the same weight. The overfed rats then increased their food intake once more, and thereafter the weight curves of both groups of rats were similar. It is unlikely that a control mechanism which was sensitive to changes in either glucose concentration or body temperature would have been able to regulate body weight over such a long time, and correct for so large an accumulated error in energy balance. To meet objections of this sort, the lipostatic theory has been put forward, and is reviewed by Kennedy[29,30]. If the total mass of fat in the animal is the factor which is monitored, then the results of Cohn and Joseph[28] can be explained. A possible mechanism by which total fat stores might be monitored has been suggested by Hervey[31]. If the hypothalmic feeding centres are sensitive to a substance such as a steroid which is soluble in fat, and if this substance is produced at a constant rate in the body and has a fixed turnover rate, then the total mass of fat in the body would tend to remain constant. Suppose, for example, that an animal increased its fat mass by forced overfeeding, then more of this steroid would be absorbed by the extra fat and less would be available to stimulate food intake. The animal would therefore eat less, and hence the fat stores would decrease, until the normal equilibrium was once more established.

It is extremely difficult to find out to what extent these postulated control mechanisms are applicable to man. As Edholm has shown, energy balance is not maintained within close limits over periods of two weeks, and as Wooley *et al.*[32] have shown both normal and obese subjects are extraordinarily poor at guessing if the meal which they have just consumed contained more or fewer calories than usual (see Chapter 4). When a control system operates with so long a time lag, and with such wide limits of tolerance, it is virtually impossible to test it out experimentally without overtaxing the goodwill of the most dedicated experimental subjects. However it is evident that in man the control system does not operate purely by adjusting energy intake, as is the case in the rat. Probably the longest-term experiments on experimental overfeeding in man have been those of the Vermont group[33] who obtained volunteers from the Vermont State Prison, who were persuaded to overeat to an extent which would increase their body weight by some 25%. This required an energy intake of about 6000-8000 kcal/day for 160 days. Although accurate measurements of energy expenditure were not made in this initial study, there is no doubt that a large proportion of the excess energy intake cannot be accounted for on the basis of any reasonable assumptions about the energy expenditure and the energy value of the increased tissue mass: in other words in this, as in other overfeeding experiments, a very large amount of the excess energy intake seems to have been lost. The controversy about 'luxuskonsumption' has raged for many years; it is constantly proposed, and refuted, that there is some mechanism by which excess calories are simply burned off as heat, thus preventing excess fat storage. It is probably a fair summary of the present situation to say that no one has proved, or disproved, the existence of luxuskonsumption in man. Much depends on exactly what is meant by the term, which is used differently by different authorities. It can certainly be said that in normal subjects an excess energy intake is not immediately and completely burned off: if this were so it would not be possible to produce experimental obesity by overfeeding normal subjects, but this is possible. Equally certainly it can be said that if normal subjects are fed, for example, 2000 kcal/day more than their normal energy requirements, they do not store an extra 2000 kcal/day as adipose tissue. It would be astonishing if they could do so, since this would be proposing, in effect, that they were able to convert dietary energy to body tissue with a conversion efficiency of 100%, which is an ideal unattainable even by the most carefully bred livestock, in which food conversion efficiency is increased as much as possible, for commercial reasons.

The metabolic response of men to overfeeding and underfeeding has been studied by Miller *et al.*[34] and Apfelbaum *et al.*[35] They have both shown that the metabolic rate responds to energy imbalance in such a way as to tend to restore energy balance. It has been proposed elsewhere that this may well be by an effect on the rate of turnover of tissue protein[10] and this has received some experimental support[36]. It has been shown that the decrease in resting metabolic rate in obese patients who are put on a reducing diet is associated with a large reduction in the rate of tissue protein turnover.

Figure 1.5 is an attempt to summarise a possible scheme for the control of energy balance in man. Energy intake is obviously determined largely by habitual diet, modified in the short term by the sensations of hunger and satiety, which arise at least partly from the activity of the hypothalamus. Appetite is a factor which also affects energy intake, and it is a sensation akin to hunger, but affected more by psychological and social factors than the state of energy balance (but see Chapter 7 for a discussion of appetite and hunger as well as a description of the hypothalmic mechanisms involved). The role of psychological factors in the aetiology of obesity is discussed in Chapter 4.

The factors which determine energy expenditure are muscular work and metabolic work. Metabolic work is the larger of the two components, and includes the energy requirements for the maintenance of ionic gradients across cell membranes, and the catabolism and synthesis of all the tissues of the body. It is proposed that while a part of this metabolic work is essential, and must continue to support life regardless of the state of energy balance, there is a part (of which tissue

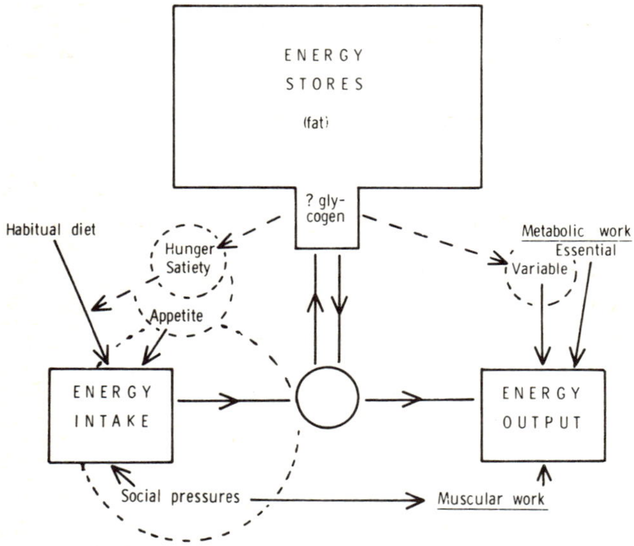

FIGURE 1.5 Possible scheme for the control of energy balance in man.

protein turnover is an example) which may proceed faster or slower depending whether there is an excessive or a deficient energy supply. This variable component of metabolic work would account for the observed changes in metabolic rate during overfeeding or underfeeding, and would contribute a fine adjustment to the mechanism for energy balance. It is indicated on the diagram that the component of energy stores from which signals originate to alter the state of hunger or satiety, or the level of the variable component of metabolic work, is the glycogen pool. This suggestion is largely speculative, but the evidence on which it is based has been set out elsewhere[10].

In obesity is the 'adipostat' broken, or set too high?

There is no doubt that in some rodents obesity is genetically determined. Bray and York[37] have written an excellent review of the various forms of genetically determined obesity in rats and mice, and they conclude that several different types of metabolic defect are involved. In all the genetically obese animals hyperphagia is a feature, but it is not possible to explain their obesity simply on the basis of overeating. For example if the ob/ob mouse is fed a restricted diet, so that its body weight is less than that of littermates fed *ad libitum*, the obese mouse will still have a greater proportion of fat in its body than the normal littermates. The metabolism of adipose tissue in obesity is the subject of Chapter 2 so this is not the place to discuss the biochemical basis for genetic obesity. The point is raised here to indicate that genetic obesity, not simply due to hyperphagia, does occur in rodents, and therefore might occur also in man. The difficulty is to know to what extent the results obtained in rodents are applicable to man. If the general outline of the control system shown in Figure 1.5 is correct, then the effect of social pressures on energy balance in man is far larger than that in a rat. Rats do not throw parties for their friends, or strive to cook appetising meals for their families. It is possible to be led far astray by assuming that the mechanism which, for example, regulates body temperature in the rat is equally relevant to man. It is true that we shiver when cold, and our hair stands up to increase the insulation of the skin, but in practice we regulate our temperature without recourse to any physiological mechanisms, and put on more clothes, or turn up the supply of heating, before the stage of shivering or goose flesh is reached. It seems quite likely that a similar situation applies with respect to energy balance: although the sensations of hunger and satiety occur in man, in practice they have relatively little influence on his food intake.

Since it is not certain how the 'adipostat' in man works, or even if it exists, it is obviously difficult to say if in obese people it is broken, or wrongly set. The argument that it is broken rests on the observation that in obese patients body weight is not well regulated, but it should be evident from the discussion above that it is not particularly well regulated in 'normal' people either. The suggestion that obese subjects have an adipostat which is set at too high a level is based largely on the premise that when obese patients are reduced in weight, they have a great tendency to relapse. Every doctor who has treated obese patients has had the experience of seeing them return some months or years later to the same weight from which the original course of treatment started. This in itself is not evidence of a physiologically 'set' weight to which the control mechanism returns. Similarly we may know individuals who have markedly reduced their cigarette smoking at some time, but who later revert to their previous practice, but this would not seriously be advanced as evidence of a physiological set point for cigarette consumption. The critical test of the set point theory is to demonstrate that there is a weight to which normal or obese people tend spontaneously to revert, and so far as I know there is no such evidence, or at least only at anecdotal level. For example Nadal *et al.*[38] reported that they knew a restaurateur in Paris who tried unsuccessfully to gain entry to the gastronomic '100 kilo club', since he could not increase his weight above 98 kg, but they provide no information about what steps he took to achieve his objective.

The best answer to the question, therefore, seems to be that there are some individuals who appear effortlessly to remain within the normal range of weight for height, while others are engaged in a ceaseless, and often unsuccessful battle against obesity. To what extent these differences are genetically determined is very difficult to say, but in my opinion there is no convincing evidence that there is a set point of weight to which the physiological control system tends to revert, although there is good evidence that there are various metabolic adaptation to energy imbalance which tend to oppose large changes in the body's energy stores.

PRACTICAL STEPS IN THE PREVENTION OR CURE OF OBESITY

Since the treatment of established obesity is so difficult and disheartening it is necessary to try hard to prevent this condition. We come, therefore, to consider again Astwood's statement 'I wish to propose that obesity is an inherited disorder due to a genetically determined defect in an enzyme: in other words that people who are fat are born fat, and nothing much can be done about it'.

The report of Johnson *et al.*[39] is highly relevant to the question of the extent to which a genetic disposition to obesity can be influenced by nutrition. The observation by McCance[1] that the subsequent growth of rats could be influenced by their level of nutrition at the suckling phase was mentioned at the beginning of this chapter. Johnson *et al.*[39] investigated the extent to which nutritional deprivation in infancy could override the genetic tendency to obesity in the obese (fafa) Zucker rat. It had already been shown by Knittle and Hirsch[40] that the cellularity of the epididymal fat pads in normal rats could be reduced by suckling them in large litters, so the study with Zucker rats involved six treatment groups: genetically non-obese Zucker rats (Fafa) were suckled either twelve to nineteen to a mother (underfed group), eight to a mother (standard fed group) or three to four to a mother, with *ad libitum* access to a high paste food for the first five weeks (overfed group). The remaining three groups were genetically obese Zucker rats (fafa) who were similarly underfed, standard fed or overfed. After weaning all rats had access *ad libitum* to a standard stock pelleted diet. The result of this study was that up to three weeks (that is, while the feeding schedules were different) the body weight was determined by the level of nutrition and not the genotype. However by twelve weeks of age, when the rats had all been on the *ad libitum* pelleted diet for nine weeks, there was a clear separation in body weight of the six groups. The three groups of genetically obese rats had all outgrown the non-obese ones, but within each genetic group there was also a clear separation according to the feeding schedule in infancy, so the overfed were heavier, and underfed lighter, than the standard fed animals, and remained so until all the animals were killed at twenty-six weeks. Thus in these rats early nutritional influences were able to modify the expression of genetic obesity, but not totally to suppress it.

It is not possible to carry out a similar study on human infants, but there is evidence that infants who are offered a formula with a high caloric density will take in more calories, and become fatter, than those who are offered the equivalent of human breast milk[41]. It has also been shown that overweight babies are more likely to become overweight children[42] and overweight adolescents tend to become overweight adults[43]. However these associations, though statistically significant, do not mean that all obese babies are predestined to eternal obesity. Melbin and Vuille[44] have analysed the relationship of obesity in infancy to overweight at school entry at the age of seven years in an entire community in Uppsala. Although there is a relationship between weight in the first year and at age seven years, as others have shown, it is not possible to predict obesity later in life from weight, or velocity of weight gain, in the first year.

It appears that it is true that, to some degree, obesity is an inherited defect, as Astwood[2] proposes, certainly in some rodents, and probably in the human species also. The nature of this defect in man is not known, and in rodents various defects have been identified. There is no justification for the view that, even if an individual has a genetic disposition to obesity, nothing can be done about it. In rats in whom there is an undoubted genetic disposition to obesity, the degree of obesity can be modified by dietary means, and there is no reason to believe that this is not so in man also. It is also evident that a great deal of obesity in man cannot be ascribed to any genetic or metabolic defect, or to an incorrect setting of the mechanism which controls body weight. The most reasonable hypothesis is that most cases of obesity occur in people who are metabolically quite normal, and who possess some capacity to regulate body weight by means of a normal hunger/satiety mechanism, and also by a normal response in metabolic rate to over- and underfeeding. However their regulating system is fairly easily overriden, so if for psychological or other reasons food intake is far in excess of requirements, there will be a steady accumulation of excess fat, not necessarily at a very high level of food conversion efficiency, which will lead eventually to obesity unless the process is interrupted. The large fluctuations in body weight which occur in the general population suggest that the mechanism which regulates body weight is often defeated, but that after a change of some 10 kg in weight, another factor, probably conscious control of food intake, comes into action, and thus body weight starts to return again to normal levels. In some people, however, this correction for large changes in weight is not made, or is not effective, and it is in these people that the problem of clinically important obesity presents.

REFERENCES

1. McCance, R. A. (1962). Food, growth and time. *Lancet*, **II**, 671
2. Astwood, E. B. (1962). The heritage of corpulence. *Endocrinology,* **71,** 337
3. Stunkard, A. and McLaren-Hume, M. (1959). The results of treatment for obesity. *Arch. Intern. Med.,* **103,** 79
4. Goldrick, R. B., Havenstein, N. and Whyte, H. M. (1973). Effect of caloric restriction and fenfluramine on weight loss and personality profile of patients with long-standing obesity. *Aust. N.Z.J. Med.,* **3,** 131
5. Davidson, S., Passmore, R. and Brock, J. F. (1969). *Human Nutrition and Dietetics,* 5th ed. (Edinburgh: Livingstone)
6. Donald, D. W. A. (1973). Mortality rates among the overweight. In *Anorexia and Obesity.* (R. F. Robertson, editor) (Edinburgh: R.C.P.)
7. Lesser, G. T., Deutsch, S. and Markofsky, J. (1971). Use of independent measurement of body fat to evaluate overweight and underweight. *Metabolism,* **20**, 792
8. Welham, W. C. and Behnke, A. R. (1942). Specific gravity of healthy men: Body weight divided by volume as an index of obesity. *J. Amer. Med. Ass.,* **118**, 498
9. Gordon, T. and Kannel, W. B. (1973). The effects of overweight on cardiovascular diseases. *Geriatrics,* **28,** 80
10. Garrow, J. S. (1974). *Energy Balance and Obesity in Man.* (Amsterdam: North Holland Publishing Co.)

11. Mitchell, H. H., Hamilton, T. S., Steggerda, F. R. and Bean, H. W. (1945). The chemical composition of the adult human body and its bearing on the biochemistry of growth. *J. Biol. Chem.,* **158**, 625
12. Widdowson, E. M., McCance, R. A. and Spray, C. M. (1951). The chemical composition of the human body. *Clin. Sci.,* **10**, 113
13. Forbes, R. M., Cooper, A. R. and Mitchell, H. H. (1953). The composition of the adult human body as determined by chemical analysis. *J. Biol. Chem.,* **203,** 359
14. Forbes, G. B. and Lewis, A. M. (1956). Total sodium, potassium and chloride in adult man. *J. Clin. Invest.,* **35,** 596
15. Wormersley, J., Boddy, K., King, P. C. and Durnin, J. V. G. A. (1972). A comparison of the fat-free mass of young adults estimated by anthropometry, body density and total body potassium content. *Clin. Sci.,* **43,**469
16. Hytten, F. E., Taylor, K. and Taggart, N. (1966). Measurement of total body fat in man by absorption of ^{85}Kr. *Clin. Sci.,* **31,** 111
17. Widdowson, E. M. and Dickerson, J. W. T. (1960). The effect of growth and function on the chemical composition of soft tissues. *Biochem. J.,* **77,** 30
18. Dickerson, J. W. T. and Widdowson, E. M. (1960). Chemical changes in skeletal muscle during development. *Biochem. J.,* **74,** 247
19. Irsigler, K., Heitkamp, H., Schlick, W. and Schmid, P. (1974). Diet and energy balance in obesity. Second Congress on energy balance in man (E. Jequier, editor) Lusanne, March 1974
20' Durnin, J. V. G. A. and Rahaman, M. M. (1967). The assessment of the amount of fat in the human body from measurement of skinfold thickness. *Brit. J. Nutr.,* **21,** 681
21. Hawes, S. F., Albert, A., Healy, M. J. R. and Garrow, J. S. (1970). A comparison of soft-tissue radiography, reflected ultrasound, skinfold calipers and thigh circumference for estimating the thickness of fat overlying the iliac crest and greater trochanter. *Proc. Nutr. Soc.,* **31,** 91A
22. Garn. S. M. (1955). Relative fat patterning: an individual characteristic. *Human Biology,* **27,** 75
23. North, K. A. K., Lascelles, D. and Coates, P. (1974). The mechanisms by which sodium excretion is increased during a fast but reduced on subsequent carbohydrate feeding. *Clin. Sci.,* **46,** 423
24. Edholm. O. G., Fletcher, J. G., Widdowson, E. M. and

McCance, R. A. (1955). The energy expenditure and food intake of individual men. *Brit. J. Nutr.,* **9,** 286

25. Mayer, J. (1970). Some aspects of the problem of regulating food intake and obesity. In *Anorexia and Obesity.* (C. V. Rowland, editor), (Boston: Little Brown and Co.), International Psychiatry Clinics, Vol. 7, No. 1, 255
26. Brobeck, J. R. (1948). Food intake as a mechanism of temperature regulation. *Yale J. Biol. Med.,* **20,** 545
27. Brobeck, J. R. (1965). *Physiological Controls and Regulation.* (W. S. Jamamoto and J. R. Brobeck, editors) (Philadelphia: Saunders)
28. Cohn, C. and Joseph, D. (1962). Influence of body weight and body fat on appetite of 'normal' lean and obese rats. *Yale J. Biol. Med.,* **34**, 598
29. Kennedy, G. C. (1953). The role of depot fat in the hypothalamic control of food intake in the rat. *Proc. Roy. Soc.* **140**, 578
30. Kennedy, G. C. (1973). Food, growth and obesity in rats. In *Energy Balance in man.* (M. Apfelbaum, editor)
31. Hervey, G. R. (1969). Regulation of energy balance. *Nature (Lond.)*, **222,**629
32. Wooley, O. W., Wooley, S. C. and Dunham, R. B. (1972). Can calories be perceived and do they affect hunger in obese and non-obese humans? *J. Comp. Physiol. Psych.,* **80,** 250
33. Sims, E. A. H., Goldman, R. F., Gluck, C. M., Horton, E. S., Kelleher, P. C. and Rowe, D. W. (1968). Experimental obesity in man. *Trans. Ass. Amer. Physicians,* **81,** 153
34. Miller, D. S., Mumford, P. and Stock, M. J. (1967). Gluttony: 2. Thermogenesis in overeating man. *Amer. J. Clin. Nutr.,* **20,** 1223
35. Apfelbaum, M., Bostsarron, J. and Lacatis, D. (1971). Effect of caloric restriction and excessive caloric intake on energy expenditure. *Amer. J. Clin. Nutr.,* **24,** 1405
36. Sender, P. M., Garlick, P. J. and James, W. P. T. (1974). Protein metabolism in obesity. Second Congress on energy balance in man (E. Jequier, editor) Lusanne, March 1974
37. Bray, G. A. and York, D. A. (1971). Genetically transmitted obesity in rodents. *Physiol. Rev.,* **51,** 598
38. Nadal, R., Nel, M. and Ravina, A. (1954). Obésité et rontgen thérapie hypophysaire. *Presse med.,* **62,** 1664
39. Johnson, P. R., Stern, S. S., Greenwood, M. R. C., Zucker, L. M. and Hirsch, J. (1974). Effect of early nutrition on adipose

cellularity and pancreatic insulin release in the Zucker rat. *J. Nutr.,* **103**, 738

40. Knittle, J. L. and Hirsch, J. (1968). Effect of early nutrition on the development of rat epididymal fat pads: Cellularity and metabolism. *J. Clin. Invest.,* **47**, 2091
41. Fomon, S. J., Thomas, L. N., Filer, L. J., Zeigler, E. E. and Leonard, M. T. (1971). Food consumption and growth of normal infants fed milk-based formulas. *Acta Ped. Scand.* Suppl., 223
42. Heald, F. P. and Hollander, R. J. (1965). The relationship between obesity in adolescence and early growth. *J. Pediatr,* **67,** 35
43. Abraham, S. and Nordseik, M. (1960). The relationship of excess weight in children and adults. *Public Health Reports,* **75**, 263
44. Mellbin, T. and Vuille, J. C. (1973). Physical development at 7 years of age in relation to velocity of weight gain in infancy with special reference to incidence of overweight. *Brit. J. Prev. Soc. Med.,* **27,** 225

2

Adipose Tissue Metabolism

John P. D. Reckless and David J. Galton

HISTORY

Past anatomists thought of fat cells as 'empty cells', the lipid being lost in fixation of the tissue, and attitudes to adipose tissue and its functions have till recently reflected this description. Adipose tissue was originally thought by physiologists to function only as an insulator and to give to the human body bouyancy in water. Its important metabolic role has only become apparent over the last fifteen years or so since the early metabolic studies reviewed by Shapiro and Wertheimer , and the studies in the human of Gellhorn and Marks[2], and Hirsch and Goldrick . Extensive review of these studies in man and animals was undertaken by Renold and Cahill[4].

TYPES OF FAT

Two types of adipose tissue are found in mammals, brown and white fat. The former's colour is mainly a reflection of the high content of cytochrome enzymes, which result in a very large capacity for oxidative metabolism. Brown fat has a high lipolytic rate though the majority of the fatty acid is not released, but metabolised within the tissue itself mostly back to triglyceride. This metabolic cycling may involve considerable energy utilisation and could contribute to heat generation in the tissue.

Brown fat has therefore a calorigenic as well as storage function. It is of importance particularly in small animals and to restore body temperature at the end of hibernation in some animals. In the human neonate brown fat is present in the mediastinum and subscapular regions at birth and provides heat and some fuel for other tissues. It is not present after this period in man, and subsequent discussion in this chapter relates to white adipose tissue. White fat does not function to a great extent as a means of heat production, but as a storage tissue. In man thermogenesis is mainly achieved by general body metabolism, and at times by muscle shivering, while body heat loss is reduced when required by peripheral vasoconstriction. Adipose tissue in these circumstances has an insulating role.

FUNCTION AND IMPORTANCE OF ADIPOSE TISSUE

Adipose tissue serves as a fuel cell, conserving fuel as triglyceride during times of feeding, and releasing glycerol and fatty acids for energy supply in times of fasting[5]. These functions of lipogenesis and lipolysis are similar to the processes of glycogenesis and glycogenolysis occuring in the liver, where excess carbohydrate in the form of glucose is stored as glycogen, while glucose is released during fasting to maintain blood glucose levels. The close similarities of these storage pathways and their control mechanisms will be discussed later in this chapter.

Triglyceride and glycogen comparisons

Triglyceride has a number of advantages over glycogen as a storage fuel[5] (Table 2.1). Large and variable amounts may be stored; the hydrophobic nature of the triglyceride heteropolymer allows closer stacking of

TABLE 2.1 *Comparison of glycogen and triglyceride, and their products as 'fuel' stores and as energy sources in the fasting and fed states*

	Glycogen	Triglyceride	
Weight in 70 kg man	150 - 400 g	7 - 10 kg	
Weight in 100 kg man	150 - 400 g	35 kg	
Energy of combustion	4.2 kcal/g	9.5 kcal/g	
Fasting blood levels	Glucose 75 mg/100 ml	Free fatty acids	60 mg/100 ml
		Triglyceride	150 mg/100 ml
		Ketones	25 mg/100 ml
Fed blood levels	Glucose 150 mg/100 ml	Free fatty acids	15 mg/100 ml
		Triglyceride	Variably raised
		Ketones	Nil
Turnover times (half-life)	Glucose 30 minutes	Free fatty acids	3 minutes
		Triglyceride	180 minutes
		Ketones	10 minutes

molecules than in the branched homopolymer of glycogen which being hydrophilic allows entrapped water (see Chapter 1); triglyceride gives a higher calorie yield per gram on combustion, partly because the glucose residues of glycogen contain more CHOH groups, which are already partly oxidised, than does triglyceride; glycogen is stored as granules while mixed triglycerides are liquid *in vivo,* mixtures of fats lowering each others melting point; and finally glycogen stores, mainly in the liver, are smaller in amount.

Disadvantages of free fatty acids as a fuel source are their relative insolubility in water and requirement for carrier sites on plasma albumin, high circulating levels of fatty acids being toxic. However, rapid turnover of blood free fatty acids result in their providing about 70-95% of fasting calorie requirements at rest and more during exercise[6]. A further disadvantage of fatty acids is that red blood cells and nervous tissue are not able to use them as a fuel source for oxidation, but require glucose. However, nervous tissue can use ketone bodies produced in the liver as partial oxidation products of fatty acids.

ADIPOSE TISSUE IN RELATION TO BODY METABOLIC STATUS

Adipose tissue is involved in the synthesis, storage and release of fuel, and it may be helpful to consider the general sequence of events in both fasting and fed states. Full reviews will be found in Galton[5], Jeanrenaud and Hepp[7], and Renold and Cahill[4].

Fasting state (Figure 2.1)

In the fasting state gut absorption of food ceases, although release from the small bowel of some very low density lipoprotein may continue. The blood levels of metabolic fuels (substrates) are maintained by the liver and adipose tissue. Glycogen is broken down to glucose, and more glucose is produced in the liver from amino acids. Lipolysis is enhanced, and free fatty acids and glycerol are released into the blood from adipose tissue, the former being carried bound to plasma albumin. Some plasma fatty acids are broken down in the liver from the more complex C_{14-20} chain to simpler water-soluble molecules. These are acetoacetate and β-hydroxybutyrate—the ketone bodies. Ketone bodies and fatty acids are taken up by the tissues, and, by a process in the mitochondria called β-oxidation, undergo chemical combustion to water and carbon dioxide. The energy released by this process is very largely coupled to other biochemical reactions, to yield 'high-energy' phosphate bonds as in adenosine triphosphate (ATP). This energy can then be coupled in turn

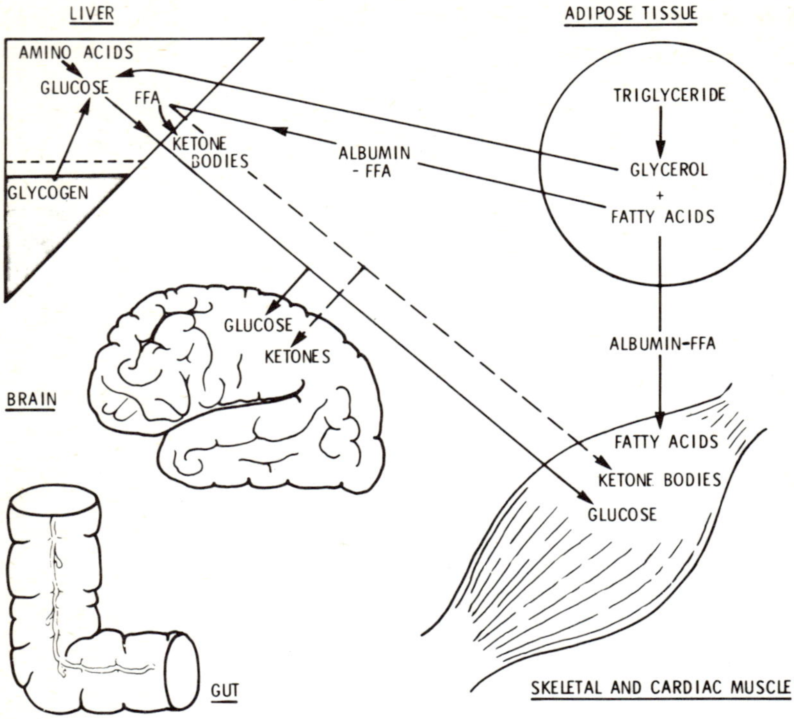

FIGURE 2.1 Blood and tissue lipid metabolism in the fasting state. The blood level of glucose is maintained by glycogenolysis and gluconeogenesis. Lipogenesis is inhibited and lipolysis enhanced, to raise the level of plasma fatty acids bound to albumin.

in a controlled manner to the essential pathways of cell metabolism, such as protein synthesis.

The glycerol, released from adipose tissue concomitantly with fatty acids from triglyceride breakdown, is also utilised, converted in the liver by gluconeogenesis to glucose. This is another mechanism by which the blood glucose in the fasting state is maintained at around 70 mg/100 ml.

Fed state (Figure 2.2)

In this situation glucose, short chain fatty acids, and amino acids are absorbed from the gut via the portal system to the liver, and fatty acids and triglycerides are passed into the blood from the lymphatics as chylomicrons. The liver replenishes its glycogen stores, and secretes very low density lipoproteins (VLDL) into the plasma. These lipoproteins consist of triglycerides and some cholesterol attached to carrier glycoprotein complexes. Adipose tissue, stimulated by the presence of insulin, removes glucose from the blood stream. At the same time fatty acids are removed from the VLDL and the chylomicrons, formed by the liver and intestine and are taken into the fat cell for triglyceride synthesis. During feeding, glucose and fatty acids continue to be utilised by many other tissues, and to a lesser extent stored in them, as glycogen granules and neutral lipid vacuoles.

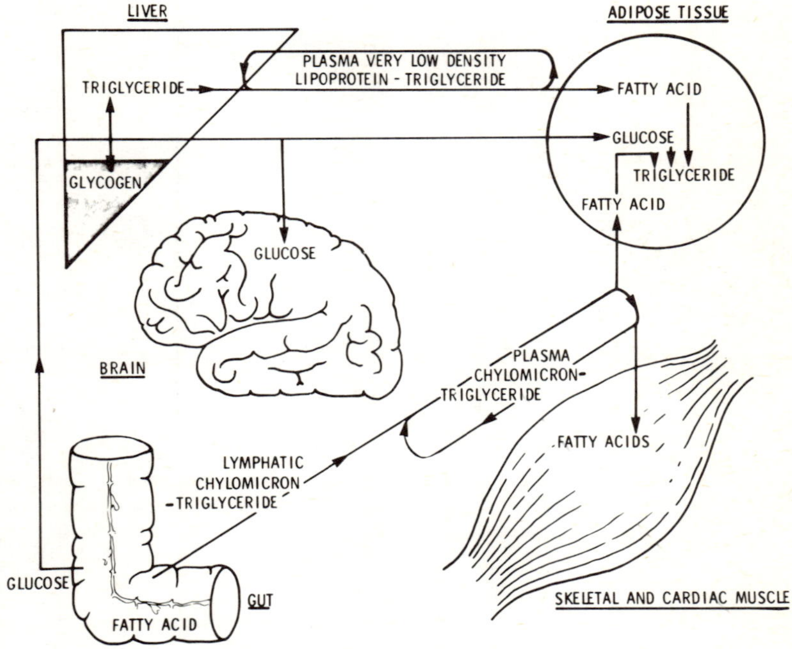

FIGURE 2.2 Blood and tissue lipid metabolism in the fed state. Fatty acids absorbed from the gut are resynthesised in the intestinal mucosa to triglyceride and secreted with lipoprotein as chylomicrons, into the lymphatics. After reaching the blood chylomicrons are hydrolysed at capillary endothelium by lipoprotein lipases. Some fatty acids are metabolised by tissues such as muscle, while the remainder are stored in adipose tissue as triglyceride. Glucose absorbed from the bowel, is partly utilised by tissue catabolism, but also is converted to glycogen and the glycerol backbone of triglyceride.

In summary then, the human body obtains most of its energy requirements during feeding from food intake, and builds up excess food into stores of glycogen and fat. In fasting the situation is reversed and fat released from adipose tissue becomes the major source of fuel for body energy requirements.

THE ROLE OF PLASMA LIPOPROTEINS IN ADIPOSE TISSUE, AND GENERAL BODY METABOLISM

A number of lipoproteins are found in normal plasma and carry various lipids which would otherwise be relatively insoluble. The lipoproteins have been classified by their physicochemical properties, by electrophoresis or in the ultracentrifuge, and carry different proportions of the various lipids (Figure 2.3), between gut, liver and the peripheral tissues.

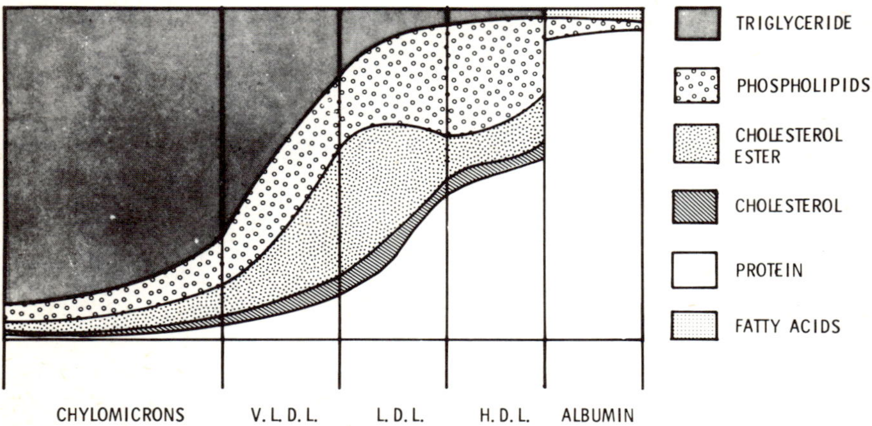

FIGURE 2.3 Relative composition of plasma lipoproteins. Lipids may be carried on a variety of protein complexes from the small albumin molecule to the very large chylomicrons. Variable proportions of each lipid type are carried on each lipoprotein group, and the relative proportions of protein and each lipid is shown in the diagram.

Dietary fat is emulsified, hydrolysed, and stabilised with lecithin, cholesterol, and conjugated bile salts to form micelles, before absorption into the small bowel mucosa. Cholesterol and bile salts are mainly reabsorbed and complete an entero-hepatic circulation. Short chain fatty acids and monoglycerides are absorbed by a simple molecular process, through the intestinal mucosa into the portal blood. The majority of hydrolysed fatty acids absorbed in the micelles are re-esterified to triglyceride in the ileal mucosa (in a similar manner to that described in adipose tissue lipogenesis). Some cholesterol is synthesised *de novo* from acetate, and together with the triglyceride and gut-synthesised lipoprotein is secreted as chylomicrons into the lymphatics. On reaching the venous blood some protein change occurs in the glycoprotein.

Most VLDL is synthesised and secreted by the liver, carrying liver-synthesised triglyceride and phospholipids. The origins and functions of the other lipoproteins, high density lipoprotein (HDL), and low density lipoprotein (LDL), are not clear, but LDL at least may be formed from VLDL when the lipid is removed from VLDL in the peripheral tissues. At least one of the subunits (apoproteins) of HDL is apparently an activator of one of the peripheral tissue lipases responsible for this lipid removal. These lipoprotein lipases are discussed later.

STRUCTURE OF ADIPOSE TISSUE

A 70 kg man has about 7-10 kg of fat in about 20-30 thousand million fat cells[5]. In obesity a very great proportion of the weight increase is in the form of stored triglyceride. A 50% increase in body weight may represent a 900% increase in adipose weight (see Chapter 1).

Changes in weight in adult life are associated with changes in fat cell size from that seen in the non-obese, of 90 ± 20 microns, while cell number remains relatively constant[8]. Some evidence suggests that overweight in intrauterine and early years of life is associated with an increased number as well as size of fat cells, and that the increased number of cells persists into adult life[8]. The evidence from animals has been extrapolated to man and it has been suggested that the increased number of cells would predispose to greater lipid accumulation and refractory obesity in some overweight adults[8]. However, other studies have suggested that in mice, cell number may increase not only in juvenile but also in adult animals[9]. In adipose tissue 60% of cells—the adipocytes—occupy nearly all the bulk of the tissue, while the remaining 40% of stromal cells are of small bulk. Some of the latter may be multipotential and become fat cells if appropriately stimulated.

Fat cell weights of triglyceride may range from 40-1000 ng, while protein content is of the order of 0.3-0.7 ng. The amount of cytosol is fairly similar in different sized fat cells, and forms a thin layer around a large central lipid droplet (Figure 2.4). It is not clear whether the lipid droplet is enclosed in a definitive protein envelope, like the protein membrane surrounding a milk drop[10]. It is clear, though, that functionally the enzymes of lipogenesis and lipolysis must be closely related to the stored lipid.

ADIPOSE TISSUE SITES

Adipose tissue is present in many parts of the body, though the extent of each site is variable, depending on age, sex, race, hormonal balance and nutritional status. Major sites are in the subcutaneous tissue of the trunk

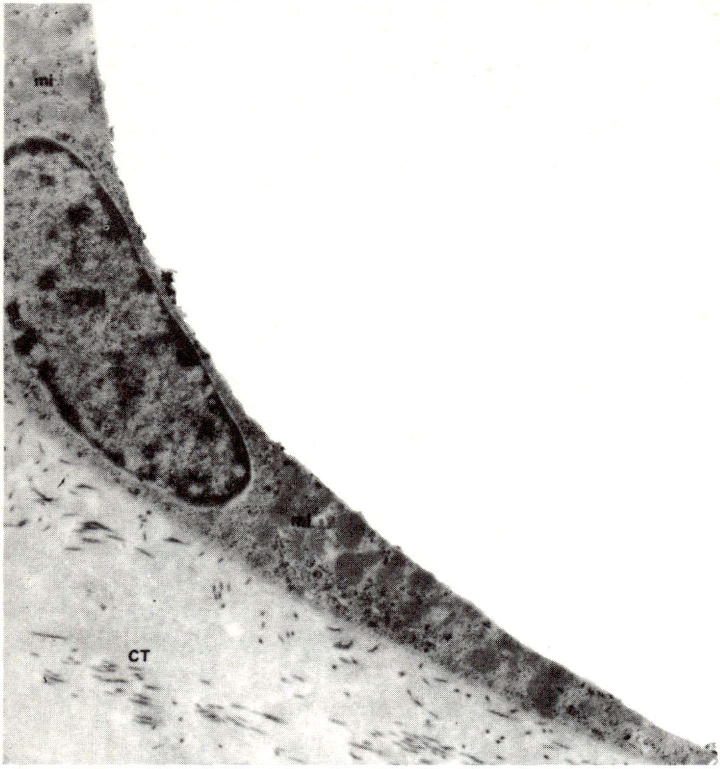

FIGURE 2.4 Electronmicrograph of part of a fat cell (x 315 000). The fat cell consists of a very large central lipid droplet surrounded by a thin rim of cytoplasm. (N= nucleus, mi= mitochondrion, CT= connective tissue).

and limb girdles, and related to thoracic and abdominal viscera, especially in the omentum and in the perinephric areas. In the female, distribution of subcutaneous fat shows increased deposition over the buttocks and thighs, and in the breasts. Some of the differences between the sexes in relation to body contour are due to variations in adiposity. Inherited factors may occasionally alter this fat deposition, with the excess fat deposition over the buttocks known as 'Hottentot bustle' or steatopygia occurring in some races, possibly being selected for as a sexual characteristic.

Sites of adipose tissue are not, however, just of anatomical interest, as there is evidence that storage and release of fuels may vary quantitatively, if not qualitatively, from site to site[8]. In addition mean cell size may vary from site to site[8].

Adipose tissue tends to accumulate as small lobules, and Bjurulf (1959) has shown that cell size decreases from the inside of the lobule outwards[11]. There are differences in function also on this basis, and Smith[12] has shown that increasing cell size is accompanied by an increase in the rate of glucose incorporation into neutral lipid.

The majority of metabolic studies in man have used abdominal subcutaneous fat biopsies. It may not always be justified to extend observations to adipose tissue from other sites, nor especially, as will become clear, to adipose tissue from other animals.

METABOLIC FUNCTIONS

As in all cells these are accomplished by chemical conversions involving many small steps allowing fine and complex controls[5]. Many of these steps have been worked out using animal tissues, and with regard to adipose tissue the rat epididymal fat pad has been most studied. Many of the pathways have been demonstrated in man, but with some qualitative and quantitative differences. Transport of materials across the cell membrane will be considered before lipogenesis and lipolysis, and hormonal effects on adipocyte metabolism.

Peripheral tissue lipid uptake

The triglyceride ultimately taken up by peripheral tissues is carried on chylomicrons and VLDL. Triglyceride is hydrolysed and fatty acid is removed from chylomicrons and the lipoproteins by the action of lipoprotein lipase (LPL) located at the vascular endothelium of the peripheral tissues (skeletal muscle, heart, and adipose tissue). LPL is probably synthesised in the peripheral tissues and secreted to the capillary endothelium. The enzyme is maximally active in adipose tissue in the fed state but the opposite occurs in muscle. Experimentally, lipoprotein lipase can be activated, and released into the blood stream, by polyanionic compounds such as heparin; though hydrolysis of triglyceride in these circumstances is probably due to activated enzyme still bound to capillary endothelium.

Several lipases (triglyceridases, phospholipases, monoglyceridases, and possibly diglyceridases) are responsible for hydrolysis of the various lipids by different tissues, rather than a single lipoprotein lipase. In Type 1 hyperlipoproteinaemia chylomicrons are not hydrolysed, and accumulate in the plasma, although the VLDL does not increase. This supports the suggestion that there are clearing factors for each lipid carrying particle. Following cleavage from circulating carriers fatty acids are transported across the cell membrane. This membrane is a complicated structure with an outer protein layer approximately 15 Å thick, and an inner mainly lipid layer 50 Å wide. The exact structure is not known but though the outer protein would be little barrier to smaller water-soluble molecules the lipid core has a complex laminar and micellar lattice structure offering a large barrier to hydrophilic molecules such as glucose. Glucose uptake is, however, an active process, stimulated by insulin, and is 10^3-10^4 greater than that expected from passive diffusion. Structural proteins in the cell membrane act as a carrier to translocate glucose and other 6-carbon sugars into (and rarely out of) the cell. Transport of fatty acids across cell membranes might involve similar active transport mechanisms.

Mitochondrial fatty acid transfer

The mechanism of fatty acid transfer across mitochondrial membranes within cells is better understood. Long chain fatty acid combined with

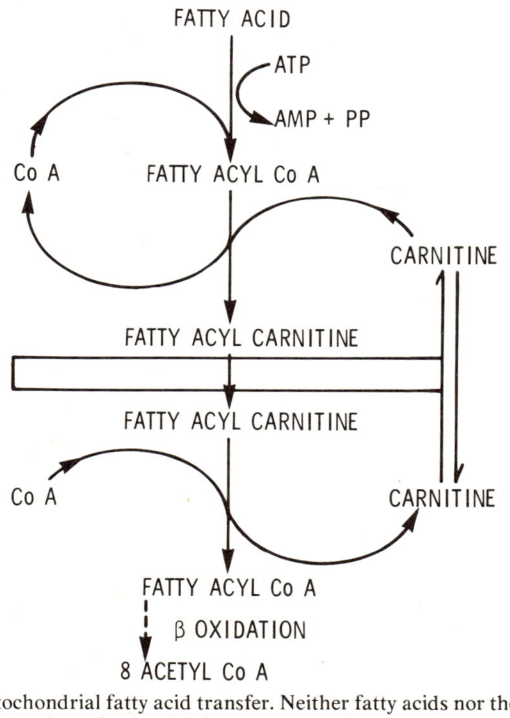

FIGURE 2.5 Mitochondrial fatty acid transfer. Neither fatty acids nor their Co-enzyme A derivatives can cross the mitochondrial membrane. However, carnitine and CoA can interchange, and the fatty acyl carnitine derivative is then able to cross the mitochondrial membrane. Within the mitochondrion fatty acyl-CoA is reformed, and the carnitine is recycled. The fatty acyl-CoA undergoes β-oxidation, and a 16-carbon fatty acid for example gives 8 acetyl-CoA groups.

Coenzyme A (fatty acyl-CoA,) is formed in cytosol, and also undergoes β-oxidation in the mitochondrion to acetyl-CoA, but cannot pass across the mitochondrial membrane. However, the fatty acyl-carnitine derivative can pass across this membrane, and the carnitine acyl transferase enzymes are present on the membrane (Figure 2.5). Fatty acyl-CoA and carnitine are reformed within the mitochondrion, the fatty acid then being able to undergo β-oxidation, while the carnitine is recycled.

Lipogenesis

Triglyceride synthesis and storage in adipocytes, or lipogenesis, involves formation of α-glycerol phosphate from glucose taken up by the cell, and the condensation on to this glycerol backbone of three activated fatty acids to give triglyceride, which is stored in the central fat droplet of the cell (Figure 2.6). The fatty acid is activated by Co-enzyme A using

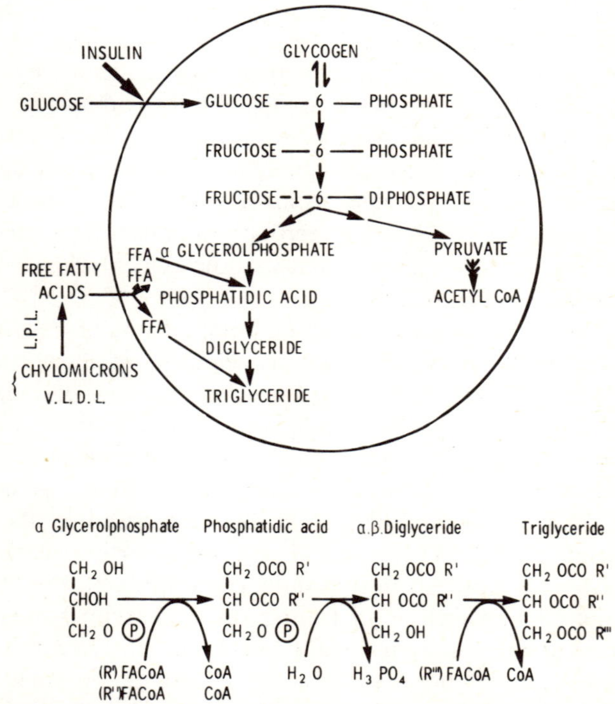

FIGURE 2.6 Outline of glycolysis and lipogenesis. Glucose is taken up by the adipocyte, especially in the presence of insulin, and is converted in a series of steps to α-glycerol phosphate. Lipoprotein lipase hydrolyses lipoprotein-triglyceride and fatty acids are taken up by the adipocyte. Two fatty acids, activated by CoA to fatty acyl-CoA, are added to the α-glycerol phosphate to give phosphatidic acid. Removal of the phosphate group gives diglyceride, and addition of a third activated fatty acid gives triglyceride.

ATP as the energy source, forming fatty acyl-CoA. The adenosine triphosphate (ATP) is generated by glycolysis and β-oxidation in the mitochondrion.

Raised plasma glucose in the fed state increases glucose uptake into tissues; and the glucose uptake is further stimulated by raised plasma insulin levels. The early part of glycolysis is probably regulated by the enzyme phosphofructokinase. Any decrease in phosphofructokinase activity will decrease glycolytic flux and lead to glucose-6-phosphate accumulation. This may itself inhibit glucose phosphorylation by hexokinase. Production of α-glycerol phosphate for lipogenesis may be regulated by the state of activity of these enzymes as well as other factors such as the NAD:NADH ratio in the cell. Some α-glycerol phosphate in the rat adipocyte may also be derived from glycerol of lipolysis. In man the appropriate enzyme, glycerolkinase, is present in small amounts, but this source of α-glycerol phosphate is thought to be unimportant[5].

The rate controlling steps in the adipocyte for fatty acid utilisation are less clearly defined at present. Activation of capillary endothelial lipoprotein lipase (LPL) is required before triglyceride on chylomicrons and VLDL is hydrolysed, while cell uptake of fatty acid may be a further step. In a fasting state it has been shown that both LPL enzyme activity and the cell uptake of fatty acid in adipose tissue from circulating lipoproteins is reduced. Further control sites exist in the chain of esterification reactions, where α-glycerol phosphate acyltransferase may be rate limiting for formation of phosphatidic acid; during fasting this enzyme is inhibited (Figure 2.6).

In some animals such as the ruminants the major results of fat digestion are smaller molecules such as acetate and short chain fatty acids. In these animals there is evidence for much *de novo* fatty acid synthesis in adipocytes from acetate, and also for chain elongation reactions to give longer chain fatty acids. While the appropriate enzymes are present in human adipose cells fatty acid synthesis is much less important than cell uptake of fatty acids synthesised in the liver or absorbed from the gut. Where subjects are fasting or in negative caloric balance, fatty acid synthesis in the adipocyte is minimal, but at times of positive caloric balance Bray (in Jeanrenaud and Hepp[7]) suggests that incorporation of glucose, pyruvate and citrate into fatty acid may occur. Goldrick and Galton[13] have recently shown that the enzymes required for fatty acid synthesis (citrate cleavage enzyme, acetyl-CoA carboxylase, and fatty acid synthetase) are all present in human adipose tissue, and that the tissue is capable of some fatty acid synthesis. However, the quantitative significance of this pathway *in vivo* has yet to be determined.

Lipolysis

Breakdown of stored neutral lipid in the adipocyte, and its release as glycerol and free fatty acids for body fuel, constitute lipolysis. The mobilisation processes are inhibited in the fed state, and activated in the fasting state. Prolonged fasting, for several days or more, may give a further rise in lipolysis, probably due to induction of new lipolytic enzymes. The other main activator of adipocyte lipolysis is hormonal stimulation. Before control mechanisms are discussed, the lipolytic enzymes should be described (Figure 2.7). These enzymes, triglyceride,

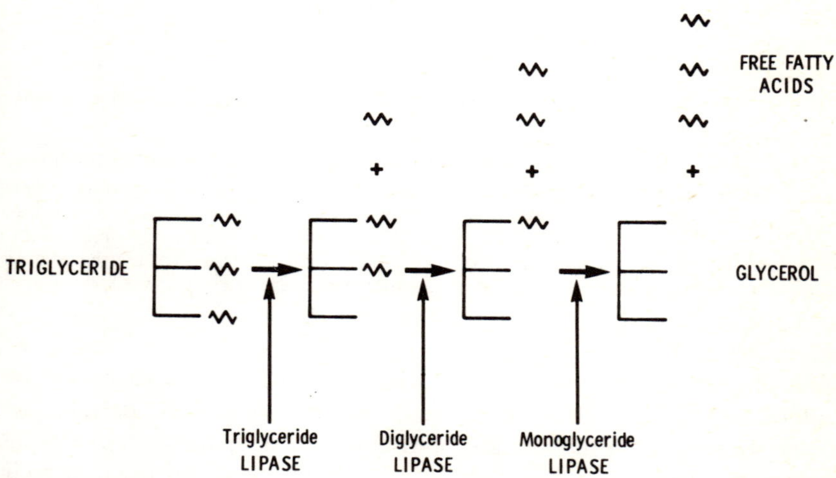

FIGURE 2.7 Lipolysis. Fatty acids are removed in turn by tri-, di-, and mono-glyceride lipases to release glycerol, and three fatty acids. The rate-limiting step is triglyceride lipase.

diglyceride and monoglyceride lipases, cleave fatty acids in turn from the glycerol backbone. The rate limiting step is triglyceride lipase upon which a controlling enzyme cascade (Figure 2.8) acts[5].

Sutherland's second messenger, the intracellular cyclic 3′5′ adenosine monophosphate (cyclic AMP)[14], is produced from ATP by the plasma membrane-bound enzyme adenyl cyclase in response to hormone stimulation (the first messenger). This sequence occurs in adipose tissue, as in many other tissues. Cyclic AMP combines with a receptor subunit of an inactive protein kinase, causing separation of receptor and catalytic subunits, the latter being the activated protein kinase. This enzyme activates in turn the triglyceride lipase by phosphorylation. This scheme of control is analogous to that modulating activity of the

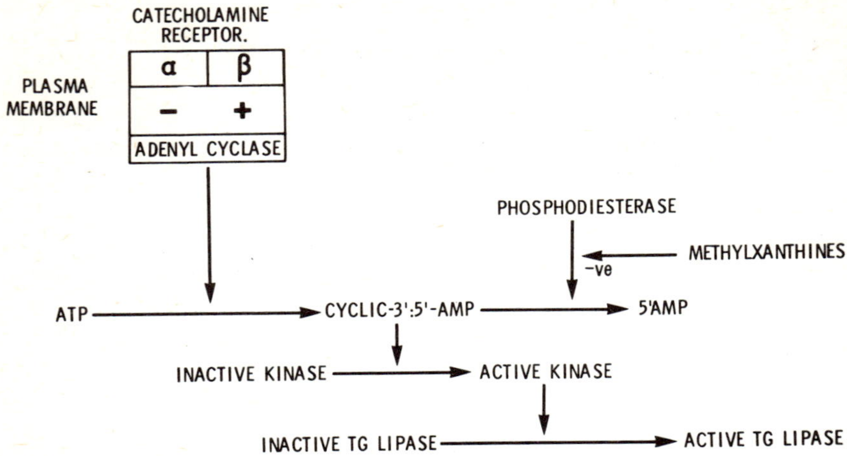

FIGURE 2.8 Controlling steps on lipolysis. Triglyceride lipase, the rate controlling step in lipolysis is activated by a series of reactions. Catecholamines have both α (inhibitory) and β(stimulatory) effects at the plasma membrane, the net effect being stimulatory. Adenyl cyclase, an enzyme bound to the inner surface of the plasma membrane is activated and cyclic AMP levels are increased. Cyclic AMP activates a protein kinase which in turn activates the lipase. Intracellular levels of cyclic AMP are reduced by the enzyme phosphodiesterase which can be inhibited by the methylxanthines.

phosphorylase for liver glycogen breakdown and this relationship will be alluded to later in the discussion of possible metabolic defects. As lipolysis and glycogenolysis are both designed to maintain circulating 'fuels' in the blood at critical levels it is perhaps not surprising that their controls should be similar.

The hormones that stimulate the adipocyte adenyl cyclase are most numerous in the rat adipocyte. These include catecholamines, ACTH, glucagon, parathormone, TSH, LH, secretin, gastrin, vasoactive intestinal peptide (VIP), vasopressin, serotonin, and possibly growth hormone and glucocorticoids. In human adipocytes only β-agonist catecholamines stimulate adenyl cyclase, the other hormones being inactive[15,16]. A further species difference here is that catecholamine α-agonist activity is inhibitory on the adenyl cyclase in man, though ineffective in rat adipocytes.

Lipolysis is inhibited by prostaglandins and insulin. Prostaglandins, especially PGE_1, are potent inhibitors, probably having their effect at the level of cyclic AMP formation. This is of interest in that it raises the possibility of an intracellular negative feedback modulating cyclic AMP formation or lipolysis. Prostaglandins could be produced during lipolysis as they are modified C_{20} fatty acids with a cyclopentane ring

(Figure 2.9). Reports of such an inhibitor have been made (Ho *et al.*)[17] but it has not been identified as a prostaglandin. An inhibitor could function *in vivo* either to limit the amount or duration of lipolysis, or to limit further cyclic AMP production once lipolysis is initiated.

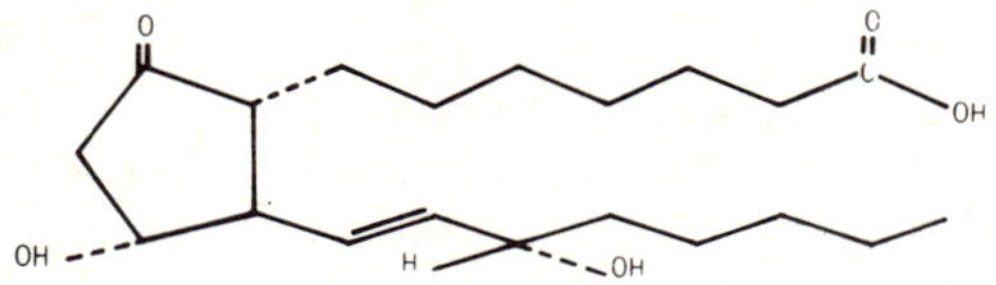

FIGURE 2.9 Structure of prostaglandin E_1. Prostaglandins are unsaturated C_{20} fatty acids modified by the presence of a cyclopentane ring.

The mode of action of insulin is not clear. In the presence of glucose increased α-glycerol phosphate formation and lipogenesis occur, while re-esterification of fatty acids may be promoted. Insulin is antilipolytic in the absence of glucose also, but in high physiological concentrations, the opposite can occur. While reduced cyclic AMP concentrations can be shown in the presence of insulin at certain concentrations and conditions in human and rat adipocytes, the changes are small and do not always correlate well with changes in lipolysis. It has not been shown convincingly whether the cyclic AMP changes are primary, and whether insulin modulates adenyl cyclase or phosphodiesterase activities.

Recent reports have raised the possibility of an insulin action through increasing the level of another intracellular cyclic nucleotide, cyclic guanosine 3'5' monophosphate (cyclic GMP)[18]. This effect is observed in one to two minutes of *in vitro* addition of insulin to adipocytes. Cyclic AMP changes, usually maximal at about five minutes may be secondary and reciprocal.

The increase in lipolysis that occurs with fasting may again be related to the fall in plasma insulin; the latter would also reduce lipogenesis. The further rise in lipolysis that occurs with prolonged fasting has been mentioned already as possibly being due to enzyme induction, but it is not clear what hormonal or intracellular stimuli are responsible for increased synthesis of the intracellular lipases. It is less likely to be due to insulin, than perhaps to growth hormone or glucocorticoid effects. Some evidence for this has been found in rat but not yet in man.

The major metabolic functions of adipocyte metabolism have been discussed in detail. In summary the triglycerides are carried either on chylomicrons from the gastrointestinal tract or on lipoproteins mainly from the liver. Lipoprotein lipase hydrolyses the triglyceride and the fatty acids can be taken up into the cells. In adipose cells glucose is also taken up and converted to α-glycerol phosphate (glycolysis). The fatty acids and α-glycerol phosphate are combined (lipogenesis) to reform triglyceride which is stored. The triglyceride may later be broken down (lipolysis) to allow release of fatty acids and glycerol. The activities of these pathways are altered by nutritional and hormonal changes.

FACTORS AFFECTING ADIPOSE TISSUE METABOLISM

Some of the hormonal effects on adipocyte metabolism have been discussed during consideration of the major pathways, but effects of the groups of hormones on these pathways will be summarised here.

Catecholamines

In human adipose tissue catecholamines have alpha (inhibitory) and beta (stimulatory) effects on lipolysis. Isoprenaline, being nearer a pure β-stimulant, is the most potent *in vitro,* and has a maximal action between 1×10^{-5} and 1×10^{-6} molar. Higher concentrations are relatively inhibitory. Noradrenaline and adrenaline have maximal *in vitro* lipolytic activity at around 1×10^{-4} molar, but are still active at or below 10^{-7} molar[16]. *In vivo* infusions[19] of these catecholamines at concentrations that may occur physiologically give marked rises in plasma free fatty acid levels. *In vitro,* both noradrenaline and adrenaline are potentiated in their effects on lipolysis by an α-blocker, such as phentolamine. Catecholamine effects on lipogenesis are indirect, and the main effects of these hormones are to increase fuel supplies to exercising muscle, and in response to stress.

The increase in free fatty acid and glycerol fuels in response to stress with physical activity is of course appropriate, but sedentary stresses may give catecholamine rises with inappropriate effects. It is recently suggested that the high plasma and myocardial free fatty acids produced by this mechanism may be toxic to an ischaemic myocardium[20]. Though this is in some dispute, the further suggestion has been made that such inappropriate effects in susceptible groups of patients may be abolished by treatment with a β-blocker, such as propranolol[21].

Insulin

Known and possible effects of insulin on adipocytes have also been partly discussed. In the fed state with raised blood glucose and insulin levels, glucose uptake, glycolysis and lipogenesis are enhanced, while lipolysis is inhibited. In the fasting state the opposite effects are noted. It is likely that the levels at which these various pathways are active, are functions of both glucose and insulin levels, and also of circulating catecholamine levels.

Prostaglandins

While prostaglandins are a specialised group of fatty acids, are synthesised in adipose tissue, and are potently antilipolytic *in vitro,* it is not clear what physiological role they play in modulating lipolysis or cyclic AMP formation.

As mentioned before, adipose tissue consists of adipocytes and stromal cells. *In vitro* low doses of prostaglandins cause cyclic AMP levels in adipose tissue to fall, but higher concentrations produce significant rises in cyclic AMP levels. The stromal cells, unlike the adipocyte, have an adenyl cyclase system which is stimulated by prostaglandins[14]. This anomaly must be remembered when interpreting prostaglandin/adipose tissues studies, which are perhaps best done in isolated fat cells separated from other cells.

Thyroid hormones

(i) Thyroid Stimulating Hormone (TSH). This hormone causes a rise in cyclic AMP levels in thyroid tissue, and also in adipose tissue (brown and white) of the rat. It is ineffective in other tissues studied, and does not have any effect in human adipose tissue[22].

(ii) Thyroxine and Tri-iodothyronine. That fat pads from hyperthyroid rats have increased sensitivity to lipolytic hormones was described by Debons and Schwartz in 1961[23]. Brodie *et al.* in 1966[24] showed that this was not due to increased lipase levels, but that increased cyclic AMP accumulation after noradrenaline stimulation occurred. Rosenqvist[25] has recently shown that the lipolytic response of adipose tissue from hypothyroid patients to noradrenaline is impaired, but that the response to noradrenaline with an α-blocker, phentolamine, is normal. Tissue from treated patients shows a normal adipocyte response to noradrenaline. It is suggested that adipose tissue in hypothyroidism shows a relatively increased α-adrenergic responsiveness to noradrenaline. This hormone has mixed α- and β-actions, and compared with normal the net lipolytic stimulus is reduced. These findings have been confirmed by our laboratory. Similar changes in cyclic AMP levels have also been shown. If replacement therapy with thyroid hormone is discontinued, the noradrenaline-stimulated cyclic AMP and glycerol increments again decrease.

Serial studies were performed on a hypothyroid patient, prior to treatment and after commencement of tri-iodothyronine (T_3) replacement. Subsequently identical placebo tablets were substituted for T_3 for a period before thyroxine (T_4) was given. Further treatment with T_3 followed. Untreated and placebo periods showed reduced lipolytic response to noradrenaline, compared with the periods on either T_3 or T_4 replacement. It is possible that thyroid hormone plays a part in maintenance or synthesis of plasma membrane, and the β-receptor part of the catecholamine receptor site might be more sensitive to thyroid lack than the α-receptor. In hyperthyroidism, serum free fatty acids may be raised in animals and man. Formation of unsaturated fatty acids from saturated fatty acids in rat liver preparations is favoured by the presence of thyroxine[26]. Low unsaturated fatty acid levels might contribute to atheroma in myxedema. In euthyroid subjects dietary deficiency of polyunsaturated fatty acids may contribute to atherosclerosis.

Other hormones

Many other hormones may affect adipose tissue metabolism in rats, but there are marked species differences, and no effects are found in human adipose tissue in acute studies. Growth hormone and glucocorticoids may be shown to have longer term actions. Other non-hormonal substances may affect fat metabolism, such as nicotinic acid which is antilipolytic, and the methylxanthines (such as caffeine and theophylline) which enhance lipolysis by competitively inhibiting phosphodiesterase (Figure 2.8).

Drugs

A number of groups of drugs may be associated with weight increase, which is often due to fluid and electrolyte changes, but may be in part due to lipid deposition. Chlorpromazine is recognised in higher doses as occasionally giving a weight increase of up to 7-10 kg, of which part may be lipid[27]. Again lithium carbonate in combination with other drugs may do the same, and amitriptyline has been similarly implicated[28]. Withdrawal of therapy is usually accompanied by loss of weight.

ADIPOSE TISSUE METABOLISM AND CONTRIBUTING FACTORS IN OBESITY

Actuarial tables provide ideal, or best-weights-for-longevity[29] and significant overweight is usually due to increased fat storage (obesity). In Chapter 1 the regulation of body weight and methods of measuring the severity of obesity are discussed. Obesity reflects a food intake over a prolonged period in excess of that required for the daily life and activities of the obese individual and requires for correction a similar period of negative caloric balance. Inactivity is clearly an important element in obesity in some patients, as Mayer[30] has documented by time lapse photography in obese adolescents. The excess food intake which can result in obesity is largely a habitual or psychogenic problem but there are other contributory factors which will be examined here.

Genetic factors in experimental animals

Genetic obesity has been described in several inbred strains of rodents, of which the ob/ob Bar Harbor obese mouse and Zucker rat are good examples. These animals inherit their disease as a Mendelian recessive, and have been compared with their lean unaffected littermates for many physiological and metabolic parameters by several groups (Bray, in Jeanrenaud and Hepp[7]). Lean unaffected littermates who had been experimentally made obese by destruction of the ventromedial nucleus of the hypothalamus (the 'satiety' centre) have also been studied.

A large number of differences may be found between lean controls and genetically obese Zucker rats but many of these are secondary to increased food intake and to the obesity that develops. Studies of adipose tissue *in vitro* show increased lipolysis and lipogenesis in the obese, but these animals also show increased food intake, high urine volumes, aberrant estrous cycles, and diminished thyroid function. The hypothalamic-lesioned controls also show some of these changes, and a hypothalamic error or lesion is probably an aetiological factor in the obesity of the Zucker rat[31].

The ob/ob mouse is, like the Zucker rat, hyperlipaemic but is also hyperglycaemic. Treble and Mayer, 1966[32], suggested that the presence of excess glycerolkinase in adipose tissue from obese mice is the principal defect, allowing rapid re-esterification and resynthesis of triglyceride. Stauffacher and Renold[33] found impaired response of muscle from obese mice to insulin, under conditions where adipose tissue remained responsive. As the obese Bar Harbor mouse is hyperinsulinaemic this possible difference in insulin sensitivities could account for many findings including decreased lipolysis, increased lipogenesis and hyperglycaemia.

Hypothalamic obesity

Mention was made in discussing genetically obese rodents of hypothalamic lesions causing obesity. In man also, damage to the ventromedial nucleus of the hypothalamus can lead to obesity. In these instances a craniopharyngioma or pituitary tumour is the usual cause, though surgical treatment of these tumours may itself lead to the hypothalamic damage. How the hypothalamus mediates the obesity and hyperphagia is not clear. Changes in pituitary hormone release are possible, while hyperinsulinaemia follows a ventromedial nucleus lesion in the rat almost immediately[34] and may be the mechanism causing obesity. In the latter study[34] Bernardis and Frohman showed that if pancreatic β-cell function was destroyed, hyperphagia and weight gain did not follow hypothalamic lesioning. Bray[31] reviews some evidence that here also hyperinsulinaemia may play a role in human hypothalamic, and perhaps general, obesity.

Genetic factors in human obesity

Genetic factors may play a part in human obesity but are much more difficult to distinguish than in laboratory animals. It is clear however, that obesity in the general population is not inherited in the simple Mendelian manner of these inbred animals, though it might yet remain to be described in further rare instances.

Metabolic obesity

Obesity in man is associated with hyperinsulinaemia, insulin resistance, and increased insulin secretion to glucose, amino acids, or tolbutamide stimuli, although glucose tolerance may be impaired. In obesity, corticosteroid secretion is increased, while growth hormone release is blunted in fasting. As in the rodents described previously these changes are probably secondary to the obesity and the increased caloric and carbohydrate diet. Studies on volunteers of normal weight before an induced weight gain, during a gain of at least 25%, and after return to basal weight have confirmed this view (Sims *et al.*[35]). The endocrine and metabolic changes observed are thus probably secondary to hyperphagia. No primary differences have been found between obese and lean groups in man to account for obesity in the majority of patients.

However, studies of the metabolic processes discussed earlier of triglyceride synthesis, storage, and release, have led recently to the observation of defects in these metabolic pathways that might favour lipid accumulation in some obese patients. Further errors in these pathways might be expected to be found as such studies continue.

Lipolytic defects

Earlier the lipolytic enzymes and the controlling enzyme system were described and the similarities with glycogenolysis noted. Glycogen and triglyceride are synthesised and stored during feeding and are released during fasting to maintain adequate blood metabolic substrate levels of glucose and fatty acids. Fall in plasma insulin levels favour release of stored 'fuel' in both cases, as does catecholamine stimulation. Various errors in the controlling enzyme system in various tissues lead to excess glycogen storage, and often present in childhood with failure to thrive and changes in the affected systems.

Similar defects in lipolysis in adipose tissue might be expected and have been provisionally classified[36] according to the site of the defect as Type I—alterations at hormone receptor or adenyl cyclase, Type II—changes at protein kinase level, and Type III—affecting the lipase. Defects in lipid handling also occur in other tissues than adipose tissue.

(i) Type I—One child who was mentally retarded at a very early age after an apparently normal full-term delivery, was born with extensive fat deposition in subcutaneous adipose tissue over feet and legs, and fingers, hands and arms, but with normal tissue proximally. After initial growth at about 10th percentile subsequent growth in weight and height over four years has been minimal, and the child now remains extremely cachectic. However, adipose deposits remain excessive peripherally, providing good clinical evidence for failure to mobilise fat from these depots. Studies at nine months of age showed no evidence of lipomatosis, and normal rates of lipogenesis from glucose and palmitate. The increment in cyclic AMP formation over basal levels in response to catecholamine stimulation, was impaired in pedal adipose tissue compared with abdominal tissue. Further, assay of cyclic AMP levels was performed by a different method three and a half years after the first studies. The basal cyclic AMP levels were found not to rise after isoprenaline stimulation of foot adipose tissue[22,36,37]. The clinical evidence for a lipolytic defect is supported by the laboratory studies, and the defect appears to be at hormone receptor or adenyl cyclase level.

(ii) Type II—An obese kindred has been described by Gilbert, Galton and Kaye[38,39], in whom three members were obese and showed impaired adipose tissue lipolysis after isoprenaline stimulation. Two of the three were also hyperlipoproteinaemic. *In vitro* adipose tissue studies also showed that cyclic AMP levels rose normally after isoprenaline stimulation. A ten-day period of fasting led to elevated plasma free fatty acid levels suggesting a triglyceride lipase normally responsive to at least one of its usual stimuli. Measured kinase activity in the adipocyte was reduced approximately 50%, but the assay was not specific for lipase kinase. Tentatively this would place the defect at the level of the protein kinase, and would be analogous to Glycogen Storage Disease Types VIII and IX which are also due to kinase defects. It is not known what proportion of lipolysis in twenty-four hours is determined by fasting, or hormonally, but obesity in this family may stem from the defect, as this would favour triglyceride deposition.

(iii) Type III—Defects in the lipase system, have not been described in adipose tissue but may yet be found and would be expected to lead to obesity. A rare lipase defect[40] has however been found in other tissues in children with Wolman's Disease[41]. Originally described as a disorder resembling Niemann Pick Disease, it is due to a lack of an acid lipase activity leading to triglyceride and cholesterol ester accumulation in viscera. As adipose tissue is apparently normal there is little lipid in the adipocyte stores, for the disorder leads to failure to thrive, cachexia, and death.

Lipogenic defects

Similarly primary defects might be expected in lipogenesis, causing increasing lipid accumulation and obesity; but have yet to be observed. With increasing obesity and increasing adipocyte size, insulin insensitivity is found but with little effect on glycolysis or lipogenesis in the adipocyte. The insulin resistance found in the ob/ob mouse has been attributed to a reduction in number[42], and possibly changes in stereochemistry, of postulated insulin receptors in various tissues. The explanation may well prove to be less simple than this.

Glycolytic defects

Lipomata are benign tumours of adipose tissue and show slow local accumulation of lipid-filled adipocytes. While some cases of multiple lipomata occur on a familial basis, nearly all lipomata are sporadic, occurring singly or in small numbers in an individual. The increasing size of a lipoma leads to some local compression of surrounding tissue, so that the tumour has distinct edges and the appearances of a capsule. It has been shown that maximal rates of lipolysis and lipogenesis are alike in tumour and control tissue, but the metabolic segment in glycolysis from fructose-6-phosphate to fructose-1-6-diphosphate (Figure 2.6) appears to be insensitive to feedback inhibition by citrate in lipomata (Atkinson *et al.*, 1974)[43]. The enzyme involved in this step, phosphofructokinase, is a complex enzyme with multiple regulatory sites[5]. The specific activity of the enzyme and response to variable ATP concentrations are similar in lipoma and normal adipose tissue. However, lack of citrate inhibition of glycolysis was demonstrated, which was also shown after extraction of phosphofructokinase from lipomata.

The especial interest of these findings is that it suggests an error of metabolic regulation of an enzyme, which may occur on an acquired rather than an hereditary basis. It may thus be distinguished from an 'inborn error', where the enzyme defect is by definition on a genetic basis. In lipoma then, glycolytic and lipogenic fluxes may at times be somewhat greater than in normal tissue, favouring excess lipid deposition in the lipoma. Whether this is the stimulus to cell division of the adipocyte precursor cell is not clear.

Endocrine factors in obesity

Corticosteroids

In obesity cortisol production rate, and twenty-four-hour urinary 17-hydroxycorticoids or 17-ketogenic steroids, are increased, but these changes are probably secondary[35]. However, the clinical picture is very similar in Cushing's syndrome where obesity is secondary. Dexamthasone suppression test will usually differentiate Cushing's syndrome and obesity. Cushing's syndrome also shows hyperinsulinaemia and often impaired glucose tolerance.

Insulinoma

This pancreatic tumour causes excessive, inappropriate insulin production, resulting in hypoglycaemia with raised plasma insulin. Symptoms of hunger and hypoglycaemia recur, while lipolysis may not be maximally activated because of raised insulin levels. The patient eats to prevent symptoms and restore blood glucose. In these circumstances the excess food intake is deposited as lipid, leading to obesity. The hyperinsulinaemia, and insulin sensitivity of simple obesity has been mentioned, as has the early hyperinsulinaemia of hypothalamic obesity. In insulinomas the raised insulin levels are primary, and MacKay *et al.*[44] have shown that gross obesity develops in normal animals given exogenous insulin. Sims' studies[35] showed that the changes in normal human volunteers overfed were secondary, so it can be concluded that, except for the rare endocrine exception, and just possibly in hypothalamic disease, the insulin changes are secondary. The evidence is more extensively reviewed by Bray *et al.*[31].

Thyroid disease

In myxoedema the basal metabolic rate is depressed in all tissues and fuel requirements are reduced. Food intake is often maintained at euthyroid levels, when weight increases. Conversely in hyperthyroidism weight usually falls, though rarely the appetite is stimulated to a greater extent than the metabolic rate, and the hyperphagia may give lipid deposition, and obesity.

Diabetes mellitus

While the juvenile insulin-dependent diabetic is usually of normal or low weight, the situation is different in the majority of obese maturity onset diabetics. They are somewhat similar to non-diabetic obese, in that insulin resistance and hyperinsulinism are present, though the latter is not sufficient to maintain normoglycaemia in the diabetic. That impaired glucose tolerance is also a feature of many obese will be remembered.

The sites of defects in the adult, maturity onset diabetic are not clear but may be in peripheral tissues such as muscle and adipose tissue as well as in the pancreas. Following a glucose load the raised plasma fatty acid level of fasting is normally rapidly suppressed; in the adult diabetic this response is slow and impaired[45]. Studies by Gilbert, Galton and Kaye[46], of adipose tissue *in vitro* showed that lipolysis is similarly inadequately suppressed by glucose loading. This may be a secondary phenomenon, but one could postulate a primary failure to suppress lipolysis leading to raised plasma free fatty acids. The fatty acids might increase plasma glucose levels by substrate competition in muscle. Both the plasma glucose, and the fatty acid levels directly, could increase insulin secretion. Lipogenesis might be favoured, especially in the presence of excess calorie intake. The glucose tolerance would be reduced by islet cell secretory failure, in the adult diabetic. Juvenile onset diabetics do not usually show evidence of peripheral tissue defects, the primary defect being pancreatic. The weight loss seen in untreated juvenile diabetics, and at times by the untreated adult diabetic, follows excessive urinary calorie loss.

Summary of contributory factors in obesity

Various factors contributing to obesity and altering adipose tissue metabolism have been discussed in this section. Genetic factors cause obesity in inbred lines of laboratory animals, and research has helped to pinpoint some of the metabolic alterations that result. Genetic factors may play some part in man but are much more difficult to elucidate. In animals and man hypothalamic damage may lead to impaired control of food intake and obesity.

Primary metabolic defects affecting the adipocyte were proposed as contributory factors in obesity, and evidence in support of some sites of defects was given. In the metabolic pathway involving the formation of α-glycerol phosphate from glucose, defective control of one of the steps may be the cause of the benign tumours, lipomata. Synthesis and subsequent breakdown of triglyceride in the fat cell (lipogenesis and lipolysis) are essential processes in body fuel regulation, and three examples of sites of defects in lipolysis are discussed. Each would favour fat deposition.

Finally in this section the alterations in hormone balance that are seen in some endocrine diseases are discussed where they favour increases in body weight.

CONCLUSIONS

Adipose tissue has been described as a fuel store used to buffer periods of fasting between intermittent food intake. Its important role in fuel homoeostasis is becoming increasingly evident after a long period of neglect which was mainly due to problems of accurate metabolic measurements. While adipocytes have all the general metabolic pathways common to cells, the processes of synthesis, storage and release of lipid have been considered in detail. Consideration of genetic, metabolic and endocrine aspects of adipose tissue metabolism have led to fresh insights into the clinical problems of obesity, lipoprotein abnormalities, and diabetes.

REFERENCES

1. Shapiro, B. and Wertheimer, E. (1956). The metabolic activity of adipose tissue—a review. *Metabolism,* **5**, 79
2. Gellhorn, A. and Marks, P. A. (1961). The composition and biosynthesis of lipids in human adipose tissues. *J. Clin. Invest.,* **41**, 925
3. Hirsch, J. and Goldrick, R. B. (1964). Serial studies on the metabolism of human adipose tissue. *J. Clin. Invest.*, **43**, 1776
4. Renold, A. E. and Cahill, G. F. Jr., editors (1965). Handbook of physiology, Section 5: Adipose tissue. *Amer. Physiol. Soc.* Washington, D.C.
5. Galton, D. J. (1971). *The Human Adipose Cell: A Model for Errors in Metabolic Regulation.* (London: Butterworths)
6. Davidson, S. and Passmore, R. (1967). *Human Nutrition and Dietetics.* (London: Livingstone)
7. Jeanrenaud, B. and Hepp, D., editors (1970). *Adipose Tissue, Regulation and Metabolic Functions.* (London: Academic Press)
8. Björntorp, P. and Östman, J. (1971). Human adipose tissue dynamics and regulation in *Advances in Metabolic Disorders.* (Levine, R. and Luft, R., editors) Vol. 5, p. 277 (London: Academic Press)
9. Lemonnier, D. (1972). Effect of age, sex and site on the cellularity of the adipose tissue in mice and rats rendered obese by a high-fat diet. *J. Clin. Invest.,* **51**, 2907

10. Dowben, R. M., Brunner, J. R. and Philpott, D. E. (1967). Studies on milk fat globule membranes. *Biochim. Biophys. Acta,* **135**, 1
11. Bjurulf, P. (1959). Atherosclerosis and body build with special reference to size and number of subcutaneous fat cells. *Acta Med. Scand.* Suppl. 349, 45
12. Smith, U. (1971). Effect of cell size on lipid synthesis by human adipose tissue *in vitro. J. Lipid Res.,* **12,** 65
13. Goldrick, R. B. and Galton, D. J. (1974). Fatty acid synthesis *de novo* in human adipose tissue. *Clinical Science and Molecular Medicine* **46,** 469
14. Robison, G. A., Butcher, R. W. and Sutherland, E. W. (1971) *Cyclic AMP.* (New York and London: Academic Press)
15. Burns, T. W., Langley, P. E. and Robison, G. A. (1971). Adrenergic receptors and cyclic AMP in the regulation of human adipose tissue lipolysis. *Annals N.Y. Acad. Sci.,* **185,** 115
16. Gilbert, C. H. and Galton, D. J. (1974). The effect of catecholamines and fasting on human adipose tissue. *Hormone and Metabolic Res.,* **46,** 469
17. Ho, R. J. and Sutherland, E. W. (1971). Formation and release of a hormone antagonist by rat adipocytes. *J. Biol. Chem.,* **246,** 6822
18. Goldberg, N. D. (1973). VIII Congress of the International Diabetes Federation. (Brussels: Excerpta Medica)
19. Harlan, W. R., Laszlo, J., Bogdonoff, M. D. and Estes, E. H. (1963). Alterations in free fatty acid metabolism in endocrine disorders. *J. Clin. End. Metab.,* **23**, 33
20. Oliver, M. F. (1973). The vulnerable myocardium. *Lancet,* 560
21. Taggart, P. and Carruthers, M. (1972). Suppression by oxprenolol of adrenergic response to stress. *Lancet,* 256
22. Reckless, J. P. D. and Galton, D. J. (1974). (Unpublished observations)
23. Debons, A. F. and Schwartz, I. L. (1961). Dependence of the lipolytic action of epinephrine *in vitro* upon thyroid hormone. *J. Lipid Res.,* **2,** 86
24. Brodie, B. B., Davies, J. I., Hynie, S., Krishna, G. and Weiss, B. (1966). Interrelationships of catecholamines with other endocrine systems. *Pharmacol. Rev.,* **18,** 273
25. Rosenqvist, U. (1972). Adrenergic receptor response in hypothyroidism. *Acta Med. Scand.* Suppl. 532
26. Faas, F. H., Carter, W. J. and Wynn, J. (1972). Effect of thyroxine

on fatty acid synthesis *in vitro. Endocrinology,* **91**, 1481
27. *Brit. Med. J.* (1974). leader, 1, 168
28. Paykel, E. S., Muelter, P. S. and de la Vergne, P. M. (1973). Amitriptyline, weight gain and carbohydrate craving: a side effect. *Brit. J. Psychiat.,* **123,** 501
29. Documenta Geigy 6th Ed. Desirable weights of adults. p. 624
30. Mayer, J. (1965). Inactivity as a major factor in adolescent obesity. *Ann. New York Acad. Sci.,* **131**, 502
31. Bray, G. A., Davidson, M. B. and Drenick, E. J. (1972). Obesity: a serious symptom. *Annals Int. Med.,* **77**, 779
32. Treble, D. H. and Mayer, J. (1963). Glycerokinase activity in white adipose tissue of obese hyperglycaemic mice. *Nature,* **200**, 363
33. Stauffacher, W. and Renold, A. E. (1969). Effect of insulin *in vivo* on diaphragm and adipose tissue of obese mice. *Amer. J. Physiol.,* **216**, 98
34. Bernardis, L. L. and Frohman, L. A. (1971). Effects of hypothalamic lesions at different loci on development of hyperinsulinaemia and obesity in the weanling rat. *J. Comp. Neurol.,* **141,** 107
35. Sims, E. A. H., Goldman, R. F., Gluck, C. M. *et al.* (1968). Experimental obesity in man. *Trans. Assoc. Amer. Physicians,* **81,** 153
36. Galton, D. J., Gilbert, C. H., Reckless, J. P. D. and Kaye, J. (1973). Triglyceride Storage Disease: a group of inborn errors of triglyceride metabolism. *Clin. Sci. Mol. Med.,* **45,** 10P
37. Kissebah, A. H., Galton, D. J., Raju, L., Kemble, M. and Scopes, J. W. (1970). (Unpublished observations)
38. Gilbert, C. H., Galton, D. J. and Kaye, J. (1973). A disorder of lipolysis in adipose tissue in two patients. *Brit. Med. J.,* **1**, 25
39. Gilbert, C. H., Galton, D. J. and Kaye, J. (1974). Proceedings of III International Congress on Regulation of adipose tissue mass. (Marseilles: Excerpta Media) p. 70
40. Kyriakides, E. C., Paul, B. and Balint, J. A. (1972). Lipid accumulation and acid lipase deficiency in fibroblasts from a family with Wolman's disease, and their apparent correction *in vitro. J. Lab. Clin. Med.,* **80**, 810
41. Wolman, M., Sterk, V. V., Gatt, S. and Frenkel, M. (1961). Primary familial xanthomatosis with involvement and calcification of the adrenals. Report of two more cases in siblings of a previously described infant. *Paediatrics,* **28**, 742
42. Kahn, C. R., Neville, D. M. Jr., Soll, A., Goldfine, I. D. and

Roth, J. (1973). Deficiency of insulin receptors in the insulin resistant obese hyperglycaemic mouse. VIII Congress of the International Diabetes Federation. (Brussels: Excerpta Medica)

43. Atkinson, J. N. C., Galton, D. J. and Gilbert, C. H. (1974). Regulatory defect of glycolysis in human lipoma. *Brit. Med. J.*, **1**, 101

44. MacKay, E. M., Callaway, J. W. and Barnes, R. H. (1940). Hyperalimentation in normal animals produced by protamine insulin. *J. Nutr.*, **20**, 59

45. Bierman, E. L., Dole, V. P. and Roberts, T. N. (1957). An abnormality of nonesterified fatty acid metabolism in diabetes mellitus. *Diabetes*, **6**, 475

46. Gilbert, C. H., Kaye, J. and Galton, D. J. (1974). The effect of a glucose load on plasma fatty acids and lipolysis in adipose tissue of obese diabetic and non-diabetic patients. *Diabetologia*, **10**, 1

3

Epidemiology of Obesity

Kateřina Ošancová and
Stanislav Hejda

In contemporary society obesity is, no doubt, a serious issue. It is studied by many specialists who are trying to resolve various aspects—from basic research into lipogenesis and lipid mobilisation to the elaboration of new reducing diets. A relatively less popular sphere is the epidemiology of obesity; obesity is no longer only the problem of individuals but of whole populations and nations.

What is the value of the epidemiological approach to obesity, how can it help to resolve or at least tackle this immense problem which already exists in many countries and is spreading to others as a by-product of civilisation? Epidemiology cannot do much to *resolve* the problem of obesity. Its main contribution is to disclose ecological and social factors which promote the development of obesity in populations, to arouse interest in its prevention and therapy and provide data which will prove the urgent need for action.

CRITERIA

Obesity means an excessive ratio of body fat, and assessment of this ratio is the only reliable method for the detection of obesity, including latent obesity, and for its classification.

However, methods which provide reliable information on the ratio of lean body mass and body fat such as hydrostatic weighing, X-ray of soft tissues, and gas dilution technique, are not suitable for epidemiological work because they are too complicated and laborious (see Chapter 1). In epidemiological work we have to be satisfied as a rule with a few objective data: body weight, height and skinfold thickness.

It is even more useful if they are supplemented by a simple physical examination, even if this is limited to visual inspection.

Body weight—The body weight should be assessed on a lever balance which is checked regularly rather than on a spring balance. Subjects should be weighed without shoes and preferably dressed only in their underwear or indoor clothes. The weights reported by the subjects themselves are rarely sufficiently reliable. Unfortunately only few epidemiological studies give an accurate account of the conditions under which the body weight was assessed.

Height—Height is usually assessed by a measuring tape and measurements should be taken without shoes.

Skinfold thickness—Assessment of skinfold thickness is a method which lends itself well to epidemiological work. Its disadvantage is that it is not very reliable and results are not readily reproducible. For measurement of the skinfold thickness various calipers are used, of which the most generally acceptable are the Harpenden type.

There are a number of sites where skinfold measurements may be taken. Keys and Brožek[1] recommended skinfold measurements at ten sites. We added two further sites—above the patella and above the coccyx (Hejda[2]). Other authors, however, measure only one skinfold, either the left subscapular or the left triceps. The latter two sites are recommended by the Committee on Nutritional Anthropometry of the National Research Council as a suitable indicator of obesity.

The number of sites and their selection depend on the type of population investigated. Obviously in investigations of representative population groups which include subjects of different ages more sites have to be used than when examining a homogeneous population group of the same sex and similar age (school children, soldiers, etc.).

From the mean subcutaneous fat layer the total amount of body fat can be calculated. Škerlj and Brožek *et al.*[3] multiply the mean subcutaneous fat layer by the body surface and index 0.94. According to Mayer[4] the subcutaneous fat accounts for *ca.* 50% of the total body fat.

Comparison of data on body fat from various authors is, however, rather difficult as the methods used differ. Some subtract from the skinfold thickness the two layers of skin (*ca.* 3 mm according to Brožek and Keys[5], Allen *et al.*[6]), others calculate the whole skinfold thickness. For the calculation of total body fat from the skinfold thickness again different procedures and formulae are used by different authors, the most recent tables are those presented by Durnin and Womersley[7]. In our experience a given formula is best suited for the group for which it was elaborated; it may be far less suitable for other groups. Skinfold thickness measurements are therefore more suited for comparison of population groups, and for longitudinal studies, where they can prove to be most valuable for recording changes over the course of time. Originally we used twelve sites in our population surveys, later we omitted those sites which correlated least with the average value of all sites, and at present measurements at eight sites are taken. These eight skinfold measurements are sufficient even for quite heterogeneous groups. Some time ago[8] we determined the sites which correlate closest with the mean, and the following sites were found most suitable for men: side of chest, hip, in younger men arm and thigh, in older men back and chest; in women: abdomen, hip, side of chest and in older women the arm.

Some authors of epidemiological surveys attempt to differentiate the type of obesity or distribution of body fat, but we feel that such distinctions go beyond the capabilities of the epidemiological approach.

In epidemiological surveys the ratio of body weight and height is used most frequently as a basis for evaluation of bodily proportions, despite the fact that this is not the most accurate method. The weight in relation to height is usually expressed as an index, although this procedure does not take into account the ratio of body fat and lean body mass nor body build or frame. Various indices have been elaborated and some are more useful than others and many are biased by the subjective views of their authors. Several of the most frequently used indices were tested and evaluated some time ago by Billewicz, Kemsley and Thomson[9] and more recently by Koshla and Lowe[10].

In the opinion of the latter authors the most suitable index is $(W^2/H) \times 100$ where W is the body weight and H the height. The correlation of this index with body weight is high and it has also other advantages.

The body weight of a subject can be evaluated also in relation to standard weights. It is, of course, important to use for this purpose national standards. The use of national standards is very useful in longitudinal studies, it has, however, the disadvantage that the findings are not comparable on an international basis.

Evaluation of the somatotype in epidemiological surveys is usually problematical regardless of whether methods based on the evaluation of photographs are used (Sheldon *et al.*[11]) or on anatomical measurements (Parnell[12]). Reliable evaluation of the somatotype is extremely difficult and laborious and in most epidemiological surveys it is not done. Despite this it is important that evaluation of recorded data should be supplemented by examination by a doctor or other specialist despite the fact that the examination may be coloured by subjective assessments. It appears that methods used by different authors and in different countries vary greatly, and are far from uniform. Moreover, the criteria of overweight and obesity used by different authors also vary. This renders difficult comparison of data published by different authors. The position would be easier if there existed an index, simple enough for epidemiological work which could express bodily proportions allowing for body frame and possibly other factors in addition.

PREVALENCE OF OBESITY

The literature on obesity and associated problems published in recent years would, no doubt, fill the bookshelves of a fair-sized library. Epidemiological studies have nevertheless been few. Therefore despite the fact that obesity is in many civilised countries one of the most widespread forms of malnutrition (Young[13]), and, no doubt, 'No condition is easier to diagnose' (Christakis[14]), our information on the prevalence of obesity in different parts of the world is still very sketchy. Nation-wide studies are extremely rare; we have to rely on information assembled in various local or regional surveys, and in groups selected according to different criteria.

Moreover, even these sketchy data are hardly comparable because of the heterogeneous character of the samples and the variable or unspecified criteria used for the assessment of overweight and obesity.

Although extremely widespread, and certainly not harmless in its consequences, obesity is not generally considered a public menace and has not been included among the notifiable diseases anywhere in the world.

With all these reservations, we have attempted to compile from the available data a mosaic of the prevalence of obesity in different countries.

Obesity in children and perspectives of childhood obesity

Paediatricians and nutritionists in many countries are concerned about the rising prevalence of obesity among children and adolescents. The majority of available data pertain, however, only to small or selected groups of children and adolescents and studies of child populations representative of different countries are extremely rare.

The Chief Medical Officer of the Ministry of Education in Great Britain[15] estimates that about 2.7% of all school children are obese. According to Börjeson[16] the prevalence of obesity among Swedish children is 2%. In the Swedish investigation obesity was roughly equally frequent in boys and girls but there were great differences among children from different socioeconomic conditions. There was more obesity among children from lower socioeconomic strata. These findings are in keeping with those of Stunkard *et al.*[17] who found that obesity was far more prevalent in lower class girls than in upper class ones—nine times as prevalent by the age of six. In boys the differences were less striking. Marchionni and Costabello[18] in Italy investigated a group comprising some 6000 six- to thirteen-year-old boys and girls and found that 5.8% were obese.

The authors of the present chapter investigated the prevalence of obesity in children and adolescents as part of a nation-wide population survey in 1971 in Czechoslovakia. Among three- to six-year-old boys it was 4%, in boys of the more advanced age groups from seven to seventeen years the prevalence of obesity varied within a very narrow range from 11.1-12.1%. The position differed in girls; while the prevalence among the youngest age group (three to six years) was negligible, it rose to 3.3% in girls aged seven to ten years. In the next two age groups the prevalence was substantially higher, 17.6% in girls aged eleven to fourteen years and 18.2% in girls fifteen to seventeen years old. Thus, as in most other studies, the prevalence of obesity among girls was found to be higher, and in the group of adolescent girls it is almost as high as in adult women of the youngest age group.

Unfortunately the data from different countries are not comparable; but even from the little we do know there is no doubt that childhood obesity is becoming an issue in industrialised countries.

In Hungary where obesity is quite frequent among adult women, Soos *et al.*[19] reported that they did not record any cases of extreme obesity in adolescents, although there was quite a proportion of adolescents who were 10-20% heavier than their ideal weight.

Beaton[20] draws attention to the increasing incidence of juvenile obesity in Canada, though he does not quote any figures. Boileau and Lizotte[21] in Canada examined more than 5000 children aged five to thirteen years and found that *ca.* 8% were obese by Mayer's criteria. Christakis[14] reports on a recent nutrition survey of 642 ten- to thirteen-year-old New York City children of whom 11% were obese.

The most extensive investigations of obesity among children and adolescents in the United States are those of Mayer's team. Thus Johnson *et al.*[22] investigated a total of 6000 youngsters and reported that 9% of the boys and 12.5% of the girls were obese.

In a more recent investigation in the United States, Dwyer *et al.*[23] recorded a 15% prevalence of obesity among adolescent girls. In

Czechoslovakia obesity in children was investigated by Luhanová[24] who found that about 10% of children in selected Prague schools were obese. She also quotes Cichecki who found in Poland that in recent years 22% of youngsters above sixteen years were obese and Vlastovski from the USSR who reports that 7% of urban children are obese.

According to numerous data adult obesity very often starts in childhood and thus there is great pressure to begin treatment and prevention of obesity at an early age.

Christakis[14] studied a large group of women and found that of 1495 white females aged twenty to sixty years 22% reported the onset of obesity before puberty, approximately 11% in their early teens, 20% after the age of twenty, 13% after marriage and 16% in association with pregnancy, only 7% became obese after the age of forty.

Bryans[25] quotes Mullins[26] who interviewed over 1000 obese adults and found that one-third were already obese during adolescence, with two-thirds developing obesity in adult life.

Asher[27] examined a group of 2000 school leavers of whom thirty-two boys and sixty-nine girls were obese. According to his data twenty-five had been obese from the age of five, sixteen of these were still obese at the age of ten and fifteen.

Heald and Hollander[28] found, in a retrospective study, that obese adolescent girls had similar birth-weights as non-obese girls. However, by the end of the first year the group who eventually became obese, had gained significantly more weight than the non-obese population. Their heights were not significantly different, nor was the mean menarchal age.

According to Brook[29] the major consequence of childhood obesity is its persistence into adult life; although it has not been established whether the prognosis differs in those children whose onset of obesity started early compared to those in whom it started later. With regard to treatment, the sooner it is started the better.

Trygstad[30], on the other hand, maintains that the prognosis regarding final weight is worst when obesity develops early. He advocates control of factors which influence adipose cell multiplication. Individuals at risk should be identified and prevention should start in the neonatal period and continue throughout life.

Most prospective studies arrived at similar conclusions. Thus Abrahams and Nordsiesk (quoted by Bryans[25]) followed up fifty overweight boys of whom 86% developed into obese adults, while only 42% of average weight boys were obese in adult life. Of fifty overweight girls 80% grew into obese adults, while only 18% average weight girls became obese in later life.

Other studies (Mayer[31]) indicate that the majority of cases of marked childhood obesity tend to persist and this is specially so in girls. According to Mayer the prognosis in obesity that starts before nine or after fifteen years is particularly poor, while obesity which develops around the puberty growth spurt is often benign and self-corrected within a few years.

Grant (quoted by Bryans[25]) in a longitudinal study of obesity comprising some 1000 children showed that a weight gain of over 10% for each 2 inches grown in height was an early sign of developing obesity specially if this trend was maintained for eight years or longer.

Some authors concerned with the perspectives of obese children have studied children from infancy. Asher[27] found that of 269 children aged eighteen months to fourteen years who were 25% or more overweight seventy-two had been obese since infancy; most of the others had become obese around the age of five.

Similar results were obtained by Eid[32] who investigated three groups of children grouped according to weight increments in the first six months of life. During check-up examinations at the age of six, seven and eight years the average weight and height was significantly higher in the children with the greatest increments during the first six months of life.

Butterfield[33] quotes June Lloyd who suggested that obese children become obese adults, and according to Smithells' experience the future prospect is gloomy. He found that scales weighing up to 20 lb are becoming useless for checking six-month-old babies, although not too long ago 20 lb was considered to be a reasonable weight for a baby approaching his first birthday.

Mellbin and Vuille[34] in Sweden, on the other hand, studied the physical development at seven years in relation to velocity of weight gain in infancy with regard to the development of obesity and concluded that their findings do not support the hypothesis that infant overnutrition is an important cause of obesity in urban Swedish children.

Although overnutrition in infancy certainly is not an irrelevant factor, it is not the only one which matters.

According to Mayer[31] a youngster has a 10% chance of being obese when his parents are of normal weight but the incidence rises to 50% when one parent is obese and to as much as 80% when both parents are obese.

While family eating habits may play a part, genetic factors are also obviously most inmportant, as is apparent from twin studies. Twins reared separately follow a similar growth pattern. When reared together, the body weight varies by *ca.* 1%, when brought up separately by about 3%.

Moreover Mayer *et al.*[31] found that obese girls differed in their somatotype from non-obese girls. The obese had a large skeleton and muscle mass, despite low activity and did not have elongated extremities.

Shukla *et al.*[35] recorded a high correlation between weight and height of obese parents and obese and overweight infants. They conclude that there may be a relationship between early nutrition and the development of infant obesity which probably is largely due to a low incidence of breast feeding and early introduction of solid foods and early weaning, as suggested by Eid[32] who investigated three groups of children classified according to weight increments in the first six months of life. During check-up examinations at the age of six, seven and eight years, he found that the mean body weight and height was significantly higher in the group of children with the highest increments in the first six months of life.

The same conclusion was reached by Taitz[36] who studied six-week-old artificially fed infants in the Sheffield region and found that they were heavier than their breast-fed counterparts. According to him this is due to intakes exceeding the classic 110 kcal/kg/day and a tendency of early feeding of solid foods. Mayer presented similar conclusions at the International Nutrition Congress in Mexico in 1972. Infants given a diet with excessive caloric density are unable to adjust to a desirable level of intake.

Several years ago a longitudinal investigation of school children was made in Czechoslovakia (Ošancová and Hejda[37]) covering a period of four to six years. At the beginning of the study the children were six to eight years old. They were divided according to their somatometric characteristics into thin, normal and obese children. 70-80% of the children remained in the original category throughout the four- or six-year period of investigation and there was not a single case where an obese child developed into a thin one or *vice versa*. Comparison of weight curves also confirmed that the weight increments per cm were higher in the obese children than in those with normal weight. The study thus supports the findings of others that the majority of individuals maintain their somatometric characteristics and that the chance that plump children will grow out of their obesity is very small. Most of the findings pertaining to the prognosis of childhood obesity thus justify prevention at a very young age.

Perhaps the clue to the problem are the results of recent work on experimental animals (Knittle and Hirsch[38]) and in man (Mayer[4]). According to these authors diet at an early age influences the number of fat cells and overnutrition leads to hyperplasia and hypertrophy of fat cells. The number of fat cells cannot be reduced by dietary restriction, only their size can be reduced. During realimentation the fat cells fill again quickly. According to Mayer a diet with excessive caloric density in infants creates conditions for hyperplasia of adipose tissue and thus a basis for future obesity.

Ashwell and Garrow[39], on the other hand, in a recent paper warn against an exaggerated fatalism as regards the supposed constancy of fat-cell number. Although, in their opinion these findings proved valuable by pointing to the importance of early nutrition, they think that this work has been misinterpreted with respect to adult obesity.

We conclude that most of the evidence suggests that the prospects of obese children 'growing out' of their excessive weight are not too hopeful. The majority of obese infants seem to grow into obese or at least overweight children who in turn are likely to develop into obese adults.

The simplest and safest way of preventing obesity in infants is breast feeding, and a return to this natural feeding in civilised countries may help to reduce the prevalence of early onset obesity.

Obesity in adults

Data on the prevalence of obesity in adults though more plentiful by far than those pertaining to children and adolescents, do not give a complete picture of the prevalence of the condition.

The number of epidemiological studies is relatively small and from many countries we possess only statistical data which pertain to small areas, or selected population groups which probably lack general validity for the whole country. Therefore any attempt to make a world-wide map of obesity is doomed to failure. The data from various countries are moreover based on different criteria of obesity and therefore are not strictly comparable.

Baird[40] reports that the incidence of obesity in the United Kingdom is not accurately known. Regional studies indicate that about half the population is overweight.

Montegriffo[41] examined employees of an industrial company and found that 60% of the men aged forty to forty-nine years had weights higher than desirable, the incidence of overweight in females aged fifty to fifty-nine years being 64%.

Comparisons with previous studies in the UK show an increase of overweight in males but not in females. According to Baird[40] regional differences in obesity may explain differences in the CHD mortality rate. Among earlier reports McMullen[42] mentions the experience of a general practitioner in England—9% of the men and 27% of the women attending his surgery were obese. His criterion of obesity was a body weight 18% above the desirable weight. Hopkins[43] reports an average of 17.4% of obese patients. Silverstone *et al.*[44] investigated 329 people in London selected at random, aged twenty to fifty-nine years, and found that 37% of the men and 49% of the women were at least 20% above their ideal weight.

Craddock[45] concludes from his own data and those of other authors in Great Britain that about half the women above thirty years are at least 10% overweight. The prevalence of obesity in adult men is lower—less than 10%.

Tran *et al.*[46] studied the body fatness of a French professional group of 4000 men aged forty-six to fifty-two years. Although they do not quote any figures on the prevalence of obesity, from the data on body fat it is apparent that some 50% of the men have more than 20.4% body fat including 25% of the men with a body fat content above 24%.

The International Cooperative Study of Cardiovascular Epidemiology (Keys *et al.*[47]) comprising large population groups from northern Europe (Finland, Netherlands—2439 men), and from southern Europe (Italy, Greece and Yugoslavia—6519) contains also some interesting data on body weights and obesity. As a criterion they used to body mass index W in kg/H^2 in metres and classified those with a body mass index less than 27 as normal and those with a body mass index above 27 as heavy men. In the latter category were 23.1% of the southern Europeans, but only 13.0% of the northern Europeans.

Epidemiological surveys in socialist countries are also scarce, although in recent years some data have become available. The problem of obesity in the USSR is discussed by Pokrovski[48] and Pokrovski *et al.*[49]. From epidemiological studies it emerges that in recent years the prevalence of obesity has greatly increased; as elsewhere it affects women in particular, starting at the age of thirty. Nogaller[50], also from the Soviet Union, reports a prevalence of 22.3% in the rural population and 28% in the urban population. Epidemiological surveys in Bulgaria revealed that on average 21.2% of the population above fourteen years are obese, in some areas the rate is however higher—as much as 31.2% (Tashev[51]). From field studies conducted in Poland it appears that 17% of adult men and 38% of women over twenty are obese (Falkiewicz *et al.*[52]). Pavel and Sdrobici estimate the prevalence of obesity in Rumanian towns as 20% of all adults, their criterion being 15-20% overweight[53].

An extensive investigation was conducted recently in the GDR (Müller *et al.*[54]) comprising some 80 000 people from different areas of the country. As the criterion of obesity they used 20% above Broca's index. Although this is a very lenient level, as admitted by the authors themselves, the recorded prevalence of obesity is very high. In rural areas 22.6% of the men and 49.1% of the women, in towns 13.6% of the men and 31.9% of the women are obese. At the Symposium on obesity in Varna in 1972 Möhr reported a mean prevalence of obesity in the GDR of 20% in men and 40% in women. Soos *et al.*[19] in Hungary found the highest prevalence of obesity with a body fat content of 30% or above in middle-aged industrial women workers, in women with sedentary occupations and in agricultural workers. Although in Czechoslovakia some major surveys were made where, among others, height and body weight were reported (Fetter *et al.*[55], Ripka[56]), little was known until recently about the prevalence of obesity in the country as a whole. Thus during an extensive investigation of blood pressure levels conducted by Ripka[56] heights and weights were also recorded in a representative population sample comprising some 12 000 people. It was found that 44.3% of the men and 58.7% of the women had a body weight above 105% of the desirable weight, 20.4% men and 37.5% of the women had body weights above 115.0% of the desirable weight and the ratio of severely obese subjects, i.e. those 25% or more overweight was 8.0% for men and 21.4% for women.

A small study was made by Doleček and Myslivеček[57] who recorded the body weights of people who were granted invalid pensions. 30.8% of the men and 60% of the women were obese and the heaviest patients were those suffering from ischaemic heart disease and hypertension.

Bürger *et al.*[58] investigated a small group of soldiers aged twenty to sixty years and found that more than 10% were overweight. They recorded the highest prevalence of obesity in the age range thirty-six to forty-six years where it was recorded in 63% of the subjects.

More complete information was obtained from two extensive surveys[59] conducted in 1956 and 1971. The prevalence of overweight (above 105% of the ideal weight), of obesity (above 115% of the ideal weight) and of severe obesity (above 125% of the ideal weight) is summarised in Tables 3.1 and 3.2 for 1956 and 1971. From the tables it is apparent that the prevalence of obesity and severe obesity is very high, especially among females. This high prevalence of obesity was recorded despite the fact that fairly lenient national standards are used for its evaluation (Hejda, Hátle[60]).

Hundley[61] in the United States estimated that the prevalence of obesity in middle-aged men and women is 30%. Goldblatt *et al.*[62] in an extensive study of social factors which influence obesity mention that obesity in the US is related to socioeconomic conditions. This phenomenon is most marked in women where 30% of women with a

TABLE 3.1 *Percentage distribution of height/weight ratio in the adult population 1956*

Group	% Desirable weight	Men	Women
Thin	-89	14.0	9.5
Normal weight	90-104	43.6	29.5
Overweight	105-114	26.0	18.6
Obese	115-124	8.8	18.1
Severely obese	>125	7.6	24.3

TABLE 3.2 *Percentage distribution of height/weight ratio in the adult population 1971*

Group	% Desirable weight	Men	Women
Thin	-89	12.9	11.4
Normal weight	90-104	33.3	24.0
Overweight	105-114	24.8	17.8
Obese	115-124	20.0	13.1
Severely obese	>125	9.0	33.7

lower socioeconomic status are obese, as compared with 16% in the middle class and 5% in the highest socioeconomic group.

Moore *et al.*[63] investigated a random sample of the white population in New York City aged twenty to fifty-nine years. Of 690 men 57.6% were overweight by 15% or more and 42.1% of 969 women were more than 27% overweight.

According to Craddock[45] the prevalence of obesity in the UK is almost equal in men and women, but a recent survey in London indicated that 20% of women compared to 15% of men were obese (Baird *et al.*[64])

Competent estimates on the prevalence of obesity in the US are found in *Nutrition Reviews* (Vol. 27/6, p. 168, 1969). If the 'desirable weight' as defined in the tables of the Metropolitan Life Insurance Company are used as a basis for comparison, about 30% of the men and 40% of the women above the age of thirty years are 20% or more above this weight. If, however, the 1959 Build and Blood Pressure Study Tables of the Society of Actuaries are used as a basis, only about 6% of the men and 11% of the women aged fifteen to sixty-nine years are overweight by 20% or more.

Since there is a high correlation between overweight and subcutaneous fat, it is safe to assume that anybody 20% or more overweight is obese and that his weight cannot be accounted for by body build. According to a conservative estimate the prevalence of obesity in men over thirty is about 20%, in women it is about 30%.

Hegsted[65] summarised the results of the Ten-State Survey and considers obesity a substantial problem. In that survey 5 - 25% adult men and 10 - 55% adult women were classified as obese. Obesity was more prevalent in black women and less prevalent in black men than in whites. Higher income was associated with more obesity in men but not in women.

Information on the prevalence of obesity in Canada is sketchy. Sinclair[66] reports that a country-wide survey of Pett and Ogilvie in 1954 indicated that 13% of the men and 23% of the women were obese by the criteria they used: all those with a weight over the 60th percentile and a skinfold thickness over 9 mm in men and 16 mm in women. Other studies give different figures but according to Sinclair[66] anyone who visited EXPO 67 in Montreal must have been aware of the problem of overweight in Canada. Beaton[67] considers overweight and obesity the most dominant form of malnutrition in Canada. An investigation of city employees quoted by Verdy[68] revealed a 35% prevalence of obesity in a group of men aged forty-three years.

Johnson[69] reports on a detailed study conducted in the urban population of Lagos, capital of Nigeria. The study comprised more than 900 subjects aged fifteen to sixty-four years. As a criterion of overweight, 10% above the standard weight was used. The 20% or more above standard weight were classified as obese. Of the males 4.3% were overweight and 3.1% were obese. The highest prevalence of overweight and obesity was in the age group of thirty-five to forty-four years. There was no significant difference in the prevalence of overweight and obesity in men aged fifteen to twenty-four and twenty-five to thirty-four years, nor was there a significant difference in the prevalence of overweight and obesity among men aged forty-five to fifty-four years and the subsequent decade fifty-five to sixty-four years. Overweight and obesity was much more common among females, 26.5% of the women being overweight and 14.9% obese. The highest rates of obesity were recorded in females aged fifty-five to sixty-four years—41.9% overweight and 29.0% obese.

Two surveys were also conducted recently in South Africa (Slome *et al.*[70] found obesity, taken as 125% or more of the US weight standards, more common in females than in males. The general prevalence of obesity in subjects over twenty years of age was 27.7%. Jackson *et al.*[71] made a survey among 600 Bantus in Cape Town. In this survey 37% were 15% or more over the ideal weights for their height.

Overweight and obesity seems to be less common in Nigerians from Lagos than in other African groups and certainly far less common than in Western countries.

Our world-wide map of obesity unfortunately is very incomplete. But even these incomplete data leave no doubt that obesity is becoming a real issue in advanced countries. Obesity is certainly not merely a cosmetic problem. Although its impact on health is not fully understood, as will be shown later, there certainly exists a close association between obesity and some pathological conditions. A condition which affects one-third to half the adult population in industrial countries and a fair proportion of children and adolescents deserves more attention as a public health problem than it receives at present.

Obesity in urban and rural areas

Data on the prevalence of obesity in various countries are, as mentioned before, rather sketchy and it is not surprising that the position is even worse as regards data on the prevalence by age, social status, region etc.

One of the most extensive surveys which provides data on regional differences in the prevalence of obesity was done in the German Democratic Republic[54]. This survey conducted in 1963-1968 comprised, as mentioned elsewhere, almost 80 000 adults. The criterion of obesity was a body weight exceeding Broca's index by 20% or more. When this criterion was used, the prevalence of obesity in the general population was on average 19.2% in men and 42.2% in women.

There were, however, great differences in the prevalence of obesity between towns and rural districts. The prevalence of obesity among urban men was 13.6% and in rural areas, 22.6%; the corresponding figures for women being 31.9% and 49.1%. The differences between the prevalence of obesity in urban and rural areas are striking and are similar to findings recorded in Czechoslovakia. Some findings regarding regional differences in the prevalence of obesity in Czechoslovakia are based on a nation-wide survey of blood pressure levels of the population where heights and body weights were also recorded. The total number of subjects investigated was about 12 000. The study confirmed that obesity is much more frequent in women than men and that there are considerable differences between the prevalence of obesity in the highly industrialised Western and less industrialised Eastern part of the country.

These findings give only a rough idea of the differences in the prevalence of obesity in different parts of the country and more insight into the problem can be obtained from more detailed field surveys. Findings recorded in the capital, Prague, and among representative population groups in Eastern and Western Bohemia are summarised in Table 3.3.

TABLE 3.3 *Obesity in urban and rural populations*

	% of Desirable weight			
	-104	105-114	115-124	>125
Men				
Prague	48.6	30.5	16.7	4.2
Eastern Bohemia	45.2	23.5	16.3	15.0
Western Bohemia	44.6	26.8	17.9	10.7
Women				
Prague	52.6	17.9	11.6	17.9
Eastern Bohemia	28.3	19.3	13.0	39.4
Western Bohemia	25.7	20.8	13.4	40.1

As is apparent from the table, in Prague less than half the men have normal body weights or are thin, while 4.2% are severely obese, 30% overweight and 16% obese. In the two rural areas investigated in particular the ratio of severely obese men is much higher—15% and 10.7%, as compared with 4.2% in Prague.

These differences between the prevalence of obesity in town and rural areas are much more marked in women. In Prague more than half the women are thin or have a normal body weight. Almost 18% of the women suffer from severe obesity, i.e. almost one in five have a body weight by 25% or more above their desirable weight. In the two rural areas the percentage of women with a low or normal body weight is half of that in Prague, while the ratio of severe obesities is about 40%, that is more than twice as high as in Prague. Our figures on the prevalence of obesity among women in Prague may appear low as compared with data reported by Silverstone *et al.*[44] from the London area where 37% of the men and 49% of the women were classified as obese. However, the data are hardly comparable as different criteria were used.

There are, no doubt, many factors which contribute towards the observed phenomena: the rapidly advancing mechanisation of work in industry, in agriculture and in the home, a more dense network of communications and the greater availability of palatable, attractive foods. But in our opinion the lower prevalence of obesity in towns is probably due to a greater social pressure to be slim plus a higher level of health consciousness among town-dwellers. Furthermore in agricultural areas, a part is played by home produced foods such as lard, eggs and cream being readily available.

Obesity and age

It is usually maintained that the body weight at the age of twenty-five should be taken as 'ideal' and should not increase further with advancing age. However, practically all studies which have paid attention to the relationship between age and obesity reveal that obesity is becoming more frequent with advancing age and that there occurs an inflexion of this curve somewhere between the age of fifty and sixty. These studies also reveal differences between these age-obesity curves in the two sexes, and investigations which have paid attention to additional factors such as social class (Silverstone, Gordon, Stunkard[44], Penick and Stunkard[72]) disclose even more complex relations.

Silverstone *et al.*[44], and Baird *et al.*[64] found that among the London population, as has been found in New York (Moore *et al.*[63], Goldblatt *et al.*[62]), social class, sex and age were significantly related to obesity.

The prevalence of obesity among men aged twenty to twenty-nine years was only 18%, while in the oldest group aged fifty to fifty-nine it amounted to 48%. Among women the same trend is apparent, the prevalence among women being, however, higher than in men except for the youngest age group twenty to twenty-nine years where it was similar.

According to Herman[73] who studied excess weight in relation to socio-cultural characteristics the proportions of men and women who were overweight increased with age up to sixty years. Relatively fewer men sixty years old or more were overweight but the proportion of overweight women continued to increase above this age.

Müller *et al.*[74] in the German Democratic Republic found in a very extensive epidemiological study comprising almost 80 000 people that with advancing age severe forms of obesity increased, this increase being more marked in women than in men. In men this increase is less marked and moreover, similarly as in other countries (Great Britain, CSSR), the prevalence of obesity among women is higher. In the GDR the prevalence of obesity among women is double or more that in men. Müller *et al.*[74] also draw attention to the striking inflexion of the curve of prevalence of obesity, at the age of fifty. They assume that in women this inflexion is associated with the menopause or possibly the mortality rate of the obese may be higher from the sixth decade onwards.

The relationship between obesity and age as revealed by epidemiological studies at different times in Czechoslovakia (Ošancová, Hejda[59]) is illustrated in Tables 3.4, 3.5, 3.6 and 3.7 respectively. Although there are individuals who maintain a very constant body weight with

TABLE 3.4 *Percentage distribution by age of* men *in 1956*

Group	% Desirable weight	Age (years) 20-30	30-40	40-50	>50
Thin	- 89	14.0	17.1	14.1	11.0
Normal weight	90-104	59.6	48.8	31.1	47.2
Overweight	105-114	21.1	22.0	31.1	25.3
Obese	115-124	1.8	8.5	12.6	7.7
Severely obese	>125	3.5	3.6	11.1	8.8

TABLE 3.5 *Percentage distribution by age of* women *in 1956*

Group	% Desirable weight	Age (years) 20-30	30-40	40-50	>50
Thin	- 89	18.5	11.1	5.5	4.6
Normal weight	90-104	46.9	26.9	23.4	25.6
Overweight	105-114	16.1	18.5	22.7	15.1
Obese	115-124	12.3	22.2	17.2	19.8
Severely obese	>125	6.2	21.3	31.2	34.9

TABLE 3.6 *Percentage distribution by age of* men *in 1971*

Group	% Desirable weight	Age (years) 20-30	30-40	40-50	>50
Thin	- 89	25.3	7.4	6.7	12.0
Normal weight	90-104	44.0	35.3	25.3	29.4
Overweight	105-114	14.7	29.4	28.0	27.2
Obese	115-124	14.7	17.6	24.0	22.8
Severely obese	>125	1.3	10.3	16.0	8.6

TABLE 3.7 *Percentage distribution by age of* women *in 1971*

Group	% Desirable weight	Age (years) 20-30	30-40	40-50	>50
Thin	- 89	27.1	10.0	4.8	3.7
Normal weight	90-104	40.6	24.3	19.0	12.8
Overweight	105-114	12.5	34.3	16.7	12.8
Obese	115-124	11.5	10.0	16.7	13.8
Severely obese	>125	8.3	21.4	42.9	56.9

advancing age (Fox[75]), in most studies conducted so far it was found that obesity becomes more prevalent with advancing age. As Silverstone[76] points out, this results probably from a reduced calorie output which is not matched by a reduction in calorie intake. With increasing age most people take less exercise but their eating habits change only little. This weight gain is influenced also by social factors as pointed out elsewhere.

Social factors and obesity

In recent years attention was drawn by a number of workers to another factor which influences in a significant way the prevalence of obesity—social status. Thus Moore and Stunkard[66] who analysed data from a representative sample of 1660 adults in New York City revealed a striking relationship between obesity and social class. Obesity was seven times more frequent among women of the lowest social level. Among men the same relationship exists, though to a much lesser degree.

Similarly Goldblatt *et al.*[62] found that obesity was six times more common among women of low status as compared with those of high status, upwardly mobile females were less obese (12%) than downwardly mobile ones (22%).

Silverstone[76] who studied a random sample of patients from two London general practices (163 men and 181 women) found that the prevalence of obesity increased with age for both men and women. This was particularly striking in the case of women. Very few women under thirty were obese, while a considerable proportion over forty was. The proportion of those who were 'markedly' obese (i.e. 30-45% above ideal weight) or 'massively' obese (more than 45% above ideal weight) increased in social classes IV and V, as compared with social classes I-III. Again this uneven pattern of distribution was particularly noticeable among women in the sample. Taking the age and social class distribution together, obesity was proportionately more prevalent among older women of social classes IV and V than in any other sub-group.

It has been suggested that women tend to put on weight as they grow older but women in the upper social classes care more about their weight and are subject to greater social pressure to be slim. Therefore they take appropriate dietary action to correct weight gains. However some doubt has been cast on this view by the finding that women of lower social class appear to be just as aware of their obesity as upper class women. (Ashwell and Etchell[77]). Another contributing factor may be the cost of food—a tasty low-calorie diet is, no doubt, more expensive than a diet where a greater proportion of calories is supplied in the form of cereals and fat. In a subsequent study Silverstone *et al.*[44] demonstrated that social class is a powerful indicator of obesity in London as in New York where this problem was studied by Moore and Stunkard[63] and Penick and Stunkard[72]. A similar pattern emerged from the more recent study of Baird *et al.*[64]. For London women the ratio of obesity among lower class women to that in higher class women was 2:1, in New York it was 6:1. As for men, in New York a simple inverse linear relationship exists between obesity and social class when all ages are considered. In London, however, middle-class rather than lower-class men have the highest prevalence of obesity. In the London group the older lower-class men had a low prevalence of obesity which is responsible for the overall difference in the two cities. The high level of physical activity of the older lower-class men probably accounts for the lower prevalence of obesity.

Stunkard's investigations were later supplemented by data on the influence of social class on obesity and thinness in children[17]. They found that obesity was far more prevalent in the lower class girls than in those of the upper class—nine times as prevalent by the age of six. Similar, though less striking differences, were found between boys of upper and lower socioeconomic status. Thinness in girls was, as in women, more common in upper classes. Among boys as among men there were no such differences.

Herman[73] who investigated some 400 subjects attending a health maintenance clinic at Thomas Jefferson University found significant difference in the prevalence of overweight related to educational level among women. Women with less than twelve years education were more likely to be overweight than those with higher education.

Hegsted[65] quotes some findings from the Ten-State Survey in the USA. Higher income was associated with more obesity in men but not in women. Prevalence of obesity in adolescents ranged from 5-33%. Obesity in adults and children appears to be inversely related to social class and income.

INCIDENCE OF OBESITY

Data on the prevalence of obesity, although valuable as an indicator of the scope of the problem to be dealt with, do not provide any information on the development in time, i.e. on the incidence of obesity. With data on the prevalence of obesity among population groups being scarce, it is not surprising that there are even fewer data on the incidence of obesity. Most workers concerned with the epidemiology of obesity, however, assume that its prevalence is increasing. We conducted a longitudinal study in a small village and found that even after as short a period as two years the mean body weights had increased considerably, i.e. men aged thirty-five to forty-five years gained on average 2.6 kg and women aged forty-five to fifty-five years as much as 7.8 kg.

In another population survey made in a representative population sample body weights were checked after a period of eleven years. It was found that 74% of the adult men and 71% of the women had gained weight in those eleven years—the average increment in men being 7.5 kg and in women 6.4 kg. The greatest increase in both sexes occurred in the fourth decade—8.4 kg in men and 7.5 kg in women.

To obtain more complete information on the incidence of obesity, data assembled in two extensive population surveys on representative population samples made after an interval of fifteen years were compared. In Table 3.8 obesity in men and women in the two surveys is compared.

TABLE 3.8 *Percentage distribution of adult population in 1956 and 1971*

Group	% Desirable weight	Year	Men	Women
Thin	- 89	1956	14.0	9.5
		1971	12.9	11.4
Normal weight	90-104	1956	43.6	29.5
		1971	33.3	24.0
Overweight	105-114	1956	26.0	18.6
		1971	24.8	17.8
Obese	115-124	1956	8.8	18.1
		1971	20.0	13.1
Severely obese	>125	1956	7.6	24.3
		1971	9.0	33.7

The groups comprised the entire population above twenty years of age. It is apparent that in men, the most marked difference occurred in the proportion of those classified as 'obese' men; where it increased from less than 9% to 20%. This increase was mainly at the expense of men of normal weight, where a decline of approximately 13% was recorded. This means that in men, the number of subjects of normal weight declined and the number of obese subjects increased.

A more detailed analysis of the data showed that in the fifteen-year interval a shift of overweight, obesity and severe obesity towards younger age groups had occurred. The increment in men was most marked in those classified as 'obese' whereas in women the increase was most marked in those classified as 'severely obese'.

Epidemiological surveys obviously record only changes of body weight in the course of time in relation to height. As a result of a changing dietary habits and a less active life, however, at the same time undesirable changes in body composition may have occurred.

More information on the incidence of obesity in different countries along with data on changing dietary habits would provide a basis for research into obesity and other diet-conditioned diseases of civilisation.

FOOD CONSUMPTION OF THE OBESE AND NON-OBESE

Although according to popular ideas obese subjects eat much more than their thinner counterparts, this is not supported by data from the literature. Whenever the food consumption of obese subjects has been measured and compared with controls, it has been found that they do not eat more than non-obese controls and that they may even eat less. Thus Johnson *et al.*[22] studied twenty-eight obese school girls and controls and found that the caloric intake of the obese was significantly lower. Stefanik *et al.*[78] studied a group of adolescent boys and the results were similar to Johnson's. Food intakes of obese and normal adolescents were compared also by Huenemann[79] who recorded on average lower caloric intakes in obese boys and girls than in those with normal weight. Similarly Durnin *et al.*[80] found obese fourteen-year-old girls ate less than their thinner contemporaries.

What seems more serious is that the intakes of protein, calcium, iron and riboflavin tended to parallel caloric intakes and in some surveys the obese adolescents had low intakes. About half of the girls ate less than two-thirds of the recommended allowance of calcium and iron and one-sixth had low intakes of vitamins A and C. Roughly one-third of the boys consumed less than the recommended vitamin C intake, one-third had low calcium intakes and one-tenth low iron and thiamine intakes.

Hutson *et al.*[81] recorded lower caloric intakes in adults with the highest body fat content, as compared with their leaner counterparts. McCarthy[82] studied dietary intakes and physical activity in Trinidad women and also found that the intake of the obese was lower than of those with normal weight. Maxfield and Konishi[83] who compared intakes of obese and non-obese women reached similar conclusions. Rose and Williams[84] compared body weights of large and small eaters and found that the heavy eaters weighed less than the light eaters. This is also in keeping with our own results, (Ošancová[85]). Lincoln[86], in a recent study comprising 867 men, compared caloric intakes in the sub-groups classified by ponderal index and revealed that calorie consumption did not increase with increasing obesity. When the extreme groups, i.e. the least and most obese ones were compared, the caloric intake of the obese was lower. As caloric intake did not follow obesity there was, of course, a significant difference between the caloric intake, experienced in terms of body weight, of the non-obese (48.2 kcal/kg body wt.) and the most obese (32.8 kcal/kg body wt.).

Results reported recently by Ošancová and Hejda[87] are in keeping with many of the above mentioned reports. In a population study comprising 604 men and 810 women, dietary intakes of subjects with normal weight and those 25% or more above their ideal weight were compared. The caloric intake of the severely obese men and women was lower than that of the non-obese, though the differences were not significant. The same trend was observed also for the nutrient intake including calcium, iron and vitamins. The recommended intake of many nutrients is related to body weight. The question may arise whether the obese with a much lower intake of nutrients per kg of body weight were not deficient in some vital nutrients.

More controversial than views on food intake of obese and non-obese subjects are those on the role of inactivity in the development of obesity.

As, no doubt, the physiological cost of all activities is closely related to body weight, Passmore[88] concludes that heaviness in some way diminishes physical activity. Thus fat people would be leisurely people rather than gluttons.

His view is supported by the findings of Dorris and Stunkard[89], who using pedometers, compared obese and non-obese women and found that the latter covered each day more miles than their obese counterparts. Similar results were recorded by Chirico and Stunkard[90]. Bloom and Eidex[91] compared lean and obese housewives and found that the lean women were much more active.

Bullen *et al.*[92] concluded from motion picture studies among adolescent girls that obese girls spend less energy than the non-obese. The conclusions of Stefanik *et al.*[78] for boys are similar.

Bradfield and Jourdan[93] in a recent study assessed energy expenditure during weight loss in a group of women and concluded that the obese were highly inactive. Weight loss induced by dietary means was not associated with an increased energy expenditure or increased efficiency of oxygen utilisation.

McCarthy[94], on the other hand, did not record any difference in the energy output of obese and non-obese women in Trinidad. Maxfield and Konishi[83] who compared energy outputs by using pedometers reached similar conclusions as McCarthy.

Miller and Mumford [95] do not consider overeating and inactivity the primary causes of obesity, and maintain that other factors responsible for the development of obesity must be sought.

Lincoln[86] found in his study a direct relationship between food intake and activity levels and submits the hypothesis that, if in some groups obesity leads to extreme food restriction, it may also reduce activity levels. (For a fuller discussion of the energy relations of obese as compared with non-obese subjects see Chapter 1.)

OBESITY AS A RISK FACTOR

Obesity is, or at least is suspected to be a risk factor in many diseases. Although this problem still remains controversial, some useful information can be obtained from surveys of mortality in relation to body weight. Some years ago a relationship between body weight and mortality from diabetes and cardiovascular diseases was shown[96]. The most frequently quoted data are those assembled by the Metropolitan Life Insurance Company pertaining to some 26 000 overweight men and 25 000 overweight women aged twenty-five to sixty-four years. The per cent actual/expected deaths among the obese were on average 150% for the men (180% for those aged twenty to twenty-nine years, and 131% for those aged fifty to sixty-four years). The ratio was 142% for the moderately overweight and 179% for the markedly overweight. Among women the position was similar but there was no particular trend with age[97].

The causes of death among obese people may also reveal some information on the hazard of obesity (Table 3.9). From the data in Table 3.9 it is apparent that the presence of obesity is certainly not irrelevant as a risk factor in various diseases. This is confirmed also by numerous findings reported in the literature.

Remarkable is for instance the five-year follow-up of the incidence of ischaemic heart disease by Stamler[98] in a group of more than 1300 men aged forty to fifty-nine years. During the initial examination all lacked signs of cardiac damage. Men who had in their case-history four of the main risk factors, i.e. hypercholesterolaemia, hypertension, overweight

TABLE 3.9 *Causes of death of overweight persons aged 25-74 years*

Cause of death	Per cent actual of expected deaths among obese	
	Men	Women
Diabetes mellitus	383	372
Cirrhosis of the liver	249	147
Biliary calculi	206	284
Cardiovascular-renal disease	149	177
Cancer	97	100

Quoted from Hawkins[97]

and smoking had an incidence of 28.5% ischaemic heart disease against 2.1% among those where these risk factors were absent in the case-history.

The most extensive epidemiological study conducted so far which throws light on these problems is, the Framingham study (Kannel *et al.*[99]) covering some 5127 men and women who were followed-up for a period of over twelve years for signs of intitial development of ischaemic heart disease.

Antecedent relative weight and weight gain after the age of twenty-five years proved to be strongly related to the risk of angina pectoris and sudden death but were not associated with the development of myocardial infarction. An excess risk of angina pectoris and sudden death was found in obese men with and without elevation of blood pressure and serum cholesterol. Unless accompanied by an increase of blood pressure and serum cholesterol, obesity played a negligible role in women. Subjects with both these predisposing factors and obesity had a pronounced increase in risk, greater than that associated with either factor alone. It is also important that reduction of body weight to normal reduced the hazard of angina pectoris and sudden death.

If obesity is a risk factor, it is important to know at which level overweight begins to become dangerous. Seltzer[100] devised a 'ponderal index' (height in inches over the cube root of the weight in lb) and found that a significant excess mortality over expected mortality occurs only when the level of frank obesity is reached.

Others studied the impact of obesity on the mortality from specific diseases. Thus Comstock *et al.*[101] revealed a positive correlation between the amount of body fat and coronary heart disease.

From a review on overweight and hypertension[102] it becomes evident disease in a substantial way. The association between body weight and blood pressure is closer in women and in the very obese. In the Framingham study among hypertensive men the prevalence of obesity was 13-19%, whereas among the normotensive population only 2-4%.

A longitudinal study comprising medical records of 22 000 army officers showed that two and half times as many men in the overweight category developed sustained hypertension after the age of forty-five, as compared with the control population.

In the Framingham study the risk of developing hypertension was eight times greater in those 20% overweight than in those 10% underweight. A weight gain after the age of twenty-five years was more likely to be associated with the development of hypertension than weight gains at an earlier age. The study also confirmed that obese subjects developed diabetes, cerebrovascular disease, coronary heart disease more often than their lean counterparts. Pavel and Sdrobici[53] who studied problems of obesity in Roumania reached similar conclusions.

In Czechoslovakia as part of an epidemiological research programme focused on factors influencing the development of atherosclerosis the dietary habits and living pattern in two areas with a significant difference in the prevalence of ischaemic heart disease (IHD) (Table 3.10) were compared.

TABLE 3.10 *Prevalence and incidence of Ischaemic Heart Disease (IHD) and diet in a rural population aged 40-69 years*
(↔ $p<0.05$)

	Men			Women		
	Mountains		Lowlands	Mountains		Lowlands
Epidemiology of IHD						
Clinical prevalence % (n = 376)	11.3	↔	20.0	13.5		14.3
Morphological prevalence % (n=120)	34.1	↔	62.8	3.4		6.2
Clinical incidence % (n=527)	9.6		14.3	9.4		9.6
Diet						
Caloric intake/day	2745	↔	3139	2183	↔	2400
Fats g	97.2	↔	132.5	75.9	↔	98.0
Carbohydrate g	394.5		383.5	318.4		301.9
Protein g	77.0		89.7	60.8		69.3

The prevalence of overweight and obesity (above 110% of ideal weight) in the two areas was as follows:

	Mountains	*Lowlands*
Men	3%	42%
Women	20%	52%

In the lowland area, with the higher prevalence of IHD, obesity is much more common than in the mountains. A longitudinal study of the dietary habits in the two areas revealed moreover that in the lowland area the adverse features of the dietary habits—excessive intake of calories and fat—are becoming more accentuated, although the opposite would be desirable.

In a subsequent prospective study of ischaemic heart disease comprising 2429 people Reiniš *et al.*[103] evaluated the influence of various risk factors. They found that latent and manifest ischaemic heart disease in men as well as women increased with body weight. The greatest differences in the incidence of ischaemic heart disease were found between obese subjects and underweight subjects. The ratios were as follows (obese subjects first): men—latent IHD 13.3:3.0%, manifest IHD 10.3:6.1%. Women—latent IHD 12.8:0.0%, manifest IHD 0.4:0.0%.

Although the incidence of IHD increased with body weight, the recorded differences were not statistically significant.

Cardiovascular diseases, while being the most frequently discussed hazard of obesity, are certainly not the only one. Comstock *et al.*[101] investigated a large group of subjects and found that the mortality over a period of over fourteen years was about 12% greater for the fattest subjects. Mortality from diabetes was particularly associated with fatness; this was followed by CHD, accidents, strokes and hypertension.

Butterfield[33] draws attention to an interesting point; prevalence of diabetes in people with normal weight is 0.7%, in those 20% overweight it is 2% and in those 50% overweight it is as high as 10%.

Obesity, moreover, enhances the risk of surgical operations and anaesthesia, it causes excessive burdening of the locomotor apparatus, obese people are more liable to develop endocrine disorders, and obesity enhances the hazard of abnormal pregnancy, etc. and is also associated with psychological problems.

Data assembled on the preceding pages leave no doubt that obesity is really becoming a problem which deserves attention in many European countries and North America.

A lot has been said and written on the subject and the new facts assembled lately only confirm and expand the evidence that obesity is a disease of modern society for which a decline in physical activity and excessive intake of palatable foods with a high energy and low nutritive value are largely responsible.

The energy expenditure used for work in the majority of advanced countries is declining, and the dense network of transport facilities, public and private, are a further cause of people taking less exercise. Even housework is getting more and more mechanised. This decline of exercise ought to be compensated for by more exercise during leisure time, by sports activities, etc. However, only few people spend the energy saved at work engaging in alternative activities to expend energy—such as sports, walking, games, etc. Passmore[88] has expressed the possible future prospect most graphically: 'By the end of the twenty-first century that turbulent, bustling species *homo sapiens* may have disappeared. He may choose to evolve into *homo sedentarius,* a quiet animal who sits and uses his intelligence to pull knobs and flick switches, which control the output of atomic energy to the machines necessary to provide his food and comforts. For his leisure he may be content to rest in front of a television set or talk amiably with his neighbours. This transformation has started: if it becomes complete, then requirements for food will be cut by from one-quarter to one-third.'

The other main culprit as regards the development of obesity is the fact that in modern society highly palatable foods with a high energy and low nutritive value are plentiful and the temptation to overeat is such as to upset mechanisms for the regulation of food intake, mechanisms which in bygone times were able to maintain intake and output at the right level. Even though general agreement has not yet been reached on the harmful effect of dietary sugar, it is beyond doubt that sugar, the consumption of which has risen steeply in recent decades (in England from 15 lb per head per year in 1815 to 120 lb in 1965), has made a major contribution towards the development of obesity in many countries.

Attention should be also paid to social factors which in the light of recent research play an important part at least in some parts of the world. This will at least help to focus nutrition education on groups with the greatest risk of developing obesity.

Findings assembled in epidemiological surveys should eventually serve as a basis for programmes for the prevention of obesity. Although it will be a long way from the revelation of harmful factors and conditions which promote obesity to the prevention of its development, such an approach appears to hold the most promise. Thus far clinical efforts have proved fruitless. As Penick and Stunkard[72] pointed out most obese persons will not enter treatment; of those who do, most will not lose weight; and of those who lose weight, most will regain it.

Similar results were obtained in a survey conducted a few years ago (Ošancová, Hejda[104]) in a population with an excessive food intake and a particularly high prevalence of obesity (more than a quarter of the men and two-thirds of the women were more than 15% above their desirable weight). An attempt was made to obtain some information on the knowledge of people about the hazards of obesity and the attitude to their own body weight. The majority of the subjects (60%) were aware that obesity may cause ill health and many even had some knowledge about dietary restrictions which would help to reduce body weight. Despite this only 12% of the men and 24% of the women tried to maintain or achieve normal weights. Eight per cent of the women with normal weight wanted to put on weight and 16.5% of the severely obese (more than 25% above their desirable weight) were quite happy about their obesity and 2.2% even wanted to put on more weight.

General arguments about the adverse effects of obesity do not motivate weight reduction. Personal experience of disease, and in some groups aesthetic reasons, seem to be the most effective motivation for weight reduction.

Prevention of obesity seems worthwhile even though there is no universal agreement on all its health hazards. Some hazards are already beyond doubt, e.g. diabetes, hypertension, surgical risk, overburdening of the locomotor system, etc. and make prevention worthwhile, although the exact relationship of obesity and cardiovascular affections is not yet quite clear.

The data assembled on the perspectives of early onset obesity call not only for prevention but for prevention at an early stage. In countries with a high prevalence of obesity already, however, treatment is as urgent as prevention.

References

1. Keys, A. and Brožek, J. (1953). Body fat in adult man. *Physiol. Rev.*, **33,** 245
2. Hejda, S. (1961). Váhové a výškové charakteristiky zdravých dospělých osob se stanovením podílu podkožního tuku. *Vnitřní lék.*, **7**, 773
3. Škerlj, B., Brožek, J. and Hunt, E. E. Jr. (1953). Subcutaneous fat and age changes in body build and body form in women. *Amer. J. Phys. Anthropol.*, **11,** 577

4. Mayer, J. (1972). Symposium on obesity. IXth Intern. Congress of Nutrition, Mexico City
5. Brožek, J. and Keys, A. (1951). The evaluation of leaness fatness in man: norms and interrelationship. *Brit. J. Nutr.,* **5**, 194
6. Allen, T. H., Peng, M. T., Chen, K. B., Huang, T. F., Chang, C. and Fang, H. S. (1956). Prediction of total adiposity from skinfolds and the relationship between external and internal adiposity. *Metabolism,* **3,** 346
7. Durnin, J. V. G. A. and Womersley, J. (1974). Body fat assessed from total body density and its estimation from skinfold thickness. *Brit. J. Nutr.,* **32,** 77
8. Zvolánková, K. (1969). The importance of different sites in the assessment of the skinfold thickness by means of a caliper. VIIIth Intern. Congress of Nutrition, Prague
9. Billewicz, W. Z., Kemsley, W. F. F. and Thomson, A. M. (1962). Indices of adiposity. *Brit. J. Prev. Med.,* **16,** 183
10. Koshla, T. and Lowe, C. R. (1967). Indices of obesity derived from body weight and height. *Brit. J. Prev. Soc. Med.,* **21,** 122
11. Sheldon, W. H., Stevens, S. S. and Tucker, W. B. (1940). *The varieties of human physique.* (New York: Harper)
12. Parnell, R. W. (1958). *Behaviour and physique.* (London: Arnold)
13. Young, C. M. (1973). Overnutrition, in *Food, Nutrition, Health* (Basel: S. Karger)
14. Christakis, G. (1967). Community programs for weight reduction: Experience of the bureau of nutrition, New York City. *Canad. J. Publ. Hlth.,* **58**, 499
15. Chief Medical Officer of the Ministry of Education (1962). Report on the Health of the School Child (1960, 1961). (London: H.M.S.O.)
16. Börjeson, M. (1962). Overweight in children. *Acta Paediatr. Uppsala,* **51,** 132
17. Stunkard, A., d'Aquili, E., Fox, S. and Ross, D. L. Filion (1972). Influence of social class on obesity and thinness in children. *J. Amer. Med. Assoc.,* **221,** 579
18. Marchionni, M. and Costabello, E. (1969). Primary obesity at school age. *Minerva Pediat.,* **21,** 805
19. Soós, A. and Bouquet, D. (1971). Adatok az elhízás hazai epidemiológiájához. Data on the epidemiology of obesity in Hungary. *Egészségtudomány,* **15**, 373
20. Beaton, J. R. (1967). Energy balance and obesity. *Canad. J. Publ. Hlth.,* **58,** 479

21. Boileau, J. G. and Lizotte, P. (1972). Dépistage du nombre d'enfants obèses et étude sommaire du statut socioéconomique de leur famiłle. *Vie médicale du Canada Francaise,* **1,** 572
22. Johnson, M. L., Burke, B. S. and Mayer, J. (1957). Relative importance of inactivity and overeating in the energy balance of obese high school girls. *Amer. J. Clin. Nutr.,* **4.,** 37
23. Dwyer, J. T., Feldman, J. J. and Mayer, J. (1967). Adolescent dieters: Who are they? Physical characteristics, attitude and dieting practices of adolescent girls. *Amer. J. Clin. Nutr.,* **26,** 1045
24. Luhanová, Z. (1973). K extrémním stavům výživy u dětské populace. Sborník prací VII. konference hygieniků výživy, KHS Plzeň
25. Bryans, A. M. (1967). Childhood obesity—prelude to adult obesity. *Canad. J. Publ. Hlth.,* **58**, 486
26. Mullins, A. G. (1958). The prognosis of juvenile obesity. *Arch. Dis. Childh.,* **33,** 307
27. Asher, P. (1966). Fat babies and fat children. The prognosis of obesity in the very young. *Arch. Dis. Childh.,* **41,** 672
28. Heald, F. P. and Hollander, R. J. (1965). The relationship between obesity in adolescence and early growth. *J. Pediatr.,* **67,** 35
29. Brook, C. G. D. (1972). Consequences of childhood obesity. *World Medical Journal,* **3,** 45
30. Trygstad, O. (1972). Childhood obesity with particular reference to etiological factors. *World Medical Journal,* **3,** 49
31. Mayer, J. (1966). Some aspects of the problem of regulation of food intake and obesity. *New Engl. J. Med.,* **274,** 610, ctd. ibidem p. 662
32. Eid, E. E. (1970). Follow up study of physical growth of children who had excessive weight gain in the first 6 months of life. *Brit. Med. J.,* **2,** 14
33. Butterfield, W. J. H. (1973). Obesity—a problem in a changing world. *Nutritional Problems in a Changing World.* (D. Hollingsworth and M. Russel, editors) (London: Applied Science Publishers)
34. Mellbin, T. and Vuille, J. C. (1973). Physical Development at 7 years of age in relation to velocity of weight gain in infancy with special reference to the incidence of overweight. *Brit. J. Prev. Soc. Med.,* **27**, 225
35. Shukla, A., Forsyth, H. A., Anderson, C. M. and Marwah, S. M.

(1972). Infantile overnutrition in the first year of life: a field study in Dudley, Worcestershire. *Brit. Med. J.,* **4,** 507

36. Taitz, L. S. (1971). Infantile overnutrition among artificially fed infants in the Sheffield region. *Brit. Med. J.,* **1,** 315
37. Ošancová, K. and Hejda, S. (1964). Sledování obesity u skupin školní mládeže. *Čs. Gastroent. Výž.,* **18,** 485
38. Knittle, J. L. and Hirsch, J. (1968). Effect of early nutrition on the development of rat epididymal fat pads: cellularity and metabolism. *J. Clin. Invest.,* **47,** 2091
39. Ashwell, M. and Garrow, J. S. (1973). Full and empty fat cells. *Lancet,* **ii,** 1036
40. McLean Baird, I. (1971). Obesity and coronary heart disease. *Postgraduate Med. J.,* **47,** 30
41. Montegriffo, V. M. E. (1968). Height and weight of a United Kingdom adult population with a review of anthropometric literature. *Ann. Hum. Gen.,* **31,** 389
42. McMullen, J. J. (1959). Obesity and body weight in general practice. *Practitioner,* **182,** 222
43. Hopkins, P. (1965). Obesity in general practice. *Proc. Roy. Soc. Med.,* **58,** 197
44. Silverstone, J. T., Gordon, R. P. and Stunkard, A. J. (1969). Social factors in obesity in London. *Practitioner,* **202,** 682
45. Craddock, D. (1969). *Obesity and its management.* (Edinburgh and London: Livingstone)
46. Tran, M. H., Richard, J. L. and Lellouch, J. (1973). La graisse d'une population masculine française active des 4000 sujets de 46-52 ans. I., II. *Path. Biol.,* **21,** 747
47. Keys, A., Aravanis, C., Blackburn, H., van Buchem, F. S. P., Buzina, R., Djordjevic, B. S., Fidanza, F., Karvonen, M. J., Menotti, A., Puddu, V. and Taylor, H. L. (1972). Coronary heart disease: overweight and obesity as risk factors. *Ann. Int. Med.,* **77,** 15
48. Pokrovski, A. A. (1964). K probleme opredelenija potrebnosti čelověka v piščevyčh veščestvach. *Vestnik AMN SSR,* **19,** 3
49. Pokrovski, A. A., Bejul, E. A. and Oleneva, V. A. (1964). Dietetičeskie principi lečenia tučnosti. *Vestnik AMN SSR,* **19,** 63
50. Nogaller, A. M. and Neklejudova, E. P. (1972). Effektivnost dietoterapii bolnych ožireniem v komplexe s adipozinom ili anoreksičeskimi preparatami v ambulatornich uslovijach. Paper read at the Symposium on Obesity, Varna
51. Tashev, T. and Balabanski, L. (in press). *Diet, physical*

development and health status of the Bulgarian people. (Sofia: BAN)

52. Falkiewicz, A., Pacynski, A., Plamieniak, Z., Wojsichowsky, F. and Zawada, W. (1969). Badanie epidemiologiczne otilosci na D. Slasku. *Pol. Arch. Med Wewn.*, **42,** 3
53. Pavel, I. and Sdrobici, D. (1970). *Obezitatea.* Editura Academiei Republicii Socialiste Romania, Bucuresti
54. Müller, F. and Paul, I. (1972). Ergebnisse epidemiologischer Fettsuchtforschung in der DDR. *Ernährungsforsch.*, **17,** 237
55. Fetter, V., Titlbachová, S. and Troníček, Ch. (1956). Antropologický průzkum dospělé populace na I. celostátní spartakiádě. *Čas. Lék. Čes.*, **95,** 717
56. Ripka, O. (1968). Hypertensní nemoc. Diagnosa a léčba. SZdN Praha
57. Doleček, R. and Myslivec, V. (1967). Otylost a invalidní důchody. *Čas. Lék. Čes.*, **106,** 1366
58. Bürger, F., Klimeš, J. and Tretera, V. (1971). K otázce výskytu obesity a jejího vlivu na tělesnou výkonnost vojáků z povolání. *Voj. Zdrav. Listy,* **40**, 244
59. Ošancová, K. and Hejda, S. (1972). Incidence and prevalence of obesity in Czechoslovakia. *Nutr. Rep. International,* **6,** 191
60. Hejda, S. and Hátle, J. (1960). Váhové a výškové charakteristiky naší dospělé zdravé populace vzhledem k nutričním faktorům. *Čs. Gastroent. Výž.*, **14,**557
61. Hundley, J. M. (1955). *Weight control.* (Iowa State College Press. USA)
62. Goldblatt, P. B., Moore, M. E. and Stunkard, A. J. (1965). Social factors in obesity. *J. Amer. Med. Ass.*, **192,** 1039
63. Moore, M. E., Stunkard, A. and Srole, L. (1962). Obesity, social class and mental illness. *J. Amer. Med. Ass.*, **181,** 962
64. Baird, I. M., Silverstone, J. T., Grimshaw, J. J. and Ashwell, M. (1974). Prevalence of obesity in a London borough. *Practitioner,* **212,** 706
65. Hegsted, D. M. (1973). Nutritional surveillance in the USA. *Nutritional Problems in a Changing World.* (D. Hollingsworth and M. Russel, editors) (London: Applied Science Publishers)
66. Sinclair, D. M. (1967). Obesity as a public health problem. *Canad. J. Publ. Hlth.*, **58,** 520
67. Beaton, J. R. (1967). Energy balance and obesity. *Canad. J. Publ. Hlth.*, **58,** 479
68. Verdy, M. (1967). Obésité: mortalité et morbidité. *Canad. J. Publ. Hlth.*, **58,** 494

69. Oshotayo Johnson, T. (1970). Prevalence of overweight and obesity among adult subjects of an urban African population sample. *Brit. J. Prev. Soc. Med.,* **24,** 105
70. Slome, C., Gampel, B., Abramson, J. H. and Scotch, N. (1960). Weight, height and skinfold thickness of Zulu adults in Durban. *S. Afr. Med. J.,* **34,** 505
71. Jackson, W. P. U., Goldberg, M. D., Marine, N. and Vinik, A. I. (1968). Effectiveness, reproducibility and weight-relation of screening tests for diabetes. *Lancet,* **ii,** 1101
72. Penick, S. B. and Stunkard, A. J. (1970). Newer concepts of obesity. *Med. Clin. N. America,* **54,** 745
73. Herman, M. W. (1973). Excess weight and sociocultural characteristics. *J. Amer. Diet Ass.,* **63,** 161
74. Müller, F., Paul, I., Brasch, C., Kapell, R., v. Knorre, G., Grimmberger, E., Grimmberger, M. and Wittig, J. (1970). Zur Verbreitung der Fettsucht in der DDR. *Zt. Ges. Inn. Med. und ihre Grenzgebiete,* **25,** 1001
75. Fox. F. W. (1973). The enigma of obesity. Lancet, **ii,** 1487
76. Silverstone, J. T. (1968). Psychosocial aspects of obesity. *Proc. Roy Soc. Med.,* **61,** 371
77. Ashwell, M. and Etchell, L. (1974). Attitude of the individual to his own body weight. *Brit. J. Prevent. Soc. Med.,* **28,** 127
78. Stefanik, P. A., Heald, F. P. and Mayer, J. (1959). Caloric intake in relation to energy output of obese and non-obese adolescent boys. *Amer. J. Clin. Nutr.,* **7,** 55
79. Huenemann, R. L. (1972). Food habits of obese and non-obese adolescents. *Postgraduate Medicine,* **51,** 99
80. Durnin, J. V. G. A., Lonergan, M. E., Good, J. and Ewan, A. (1974). A cross-sectional nutritional and anthropometric study, with an interval of 7 years, on 611 adolescent school children. *Brit. J. Nutr.,* **32,** 169
81. Hutson, E. M., Cohen, N. L., Kunkel, N. D., Steinkamp, R. C., Rourke, M. H. and Walsh, H. E. (1965). Measures of body fat and related factors in normal adults. *J. Amer. Diet. Assoc.,* **47,** 179
82. McCarthy, M. C. (1966). Dietary and activity patterns of obese women in Trinidad. *J. Amer. Diet. Assoc.,* **48,** 33
83. Maxfield, E. and Konishi, F. (1966). Patterns of food intake and physical activity in obesity. *J. Amer. Diet. Assoc.,* **49**, 406
84. Rose, G. A. and Williams, R. T. (1961). Metabolic studies on large and small eaters. *Brit. J. Nutr.,* **15,** 1

85. Ošancová, K. (1961). Some results of epidemiological research into obesity. *Acta Inst. Nutr. Hum. Pragae,* **3,** 65

86. Lincoln, J. E. (1972). Calorie intake, obesity and physical activity *Amer. J. Clin. Nutr.,* **25,** 390

87. Ošancová, K. and Hejda, S. (1973). Spotřeba potravin u obézních a u osob s normální váhou. *Čs. Gastroent. Výž.,* **27,** 64

88. Passmore, R. (1962). Estimation of food requirements. *J. Roy. Statistical Soc.* Series A (General) **125,** 387

89. Dorris, R. J. and Stunkard, A. J. (1957). Physical activity: performance and attitudes of a group of obese women. *Amer. J. Med. Sci.,* **233,** 622

90. Chirico, A. M. and Stunkard, A. J. (1960). Physical activity and human obesity. *New Engl. J. Med.,* **263,** 935

91. Bloom, W. L. and Eidex, M. F. (1967). Inactivity as a major factor in adult obesity. *Metab. Clin. Exptl.,* **16,** 679

92. Bullen, B. A., Reed, R. B. and Mayer, J. (1964). Physical activity of obese and nonobese adolescent girls appraised by motion picture sampling. *Amer. J. Clin. Nutr.,* **14,** 211

93. Bradfield, R. B. and Jourdan, M. (1972). Energy expenditure of obese women during weight loss. *Amer. J. Clin. Nutr.,* **25,** 971

94. McCarthy, M. C. (1966). Dietary and activity patterns of obese women in Trinidad. *J. Amer. Diet. Assoc.,* **48,** 33

95. Miller, D. S. and Mumford, P. (1966). Obesity: Physical activity and nutrition. *Proc. Nutr. Soc.,* **25,** 100

96. Preston, T. W. and Clarke, R. D. (1966). Society of Actuaries: Build and blood pressure study. *J. Inst. Actuaries,* **92,** 27

97. Hawkins, W. W. (1963). Some medical and biological aspects of obesity. *Can. J. Publ. Hlth.,* **54,** 477

98. Stamler, J., Berkson, D. M., Young, Q. D., Hall, Y. and Miller, W. (1963). Approaches to the primary prevention of clinical coronary heart disease in high-risk middle-aged men. *Ann. N. Y. Acad. Sci.,* **97,** 932

99. Kannel, W. B., LeBauer, E. J., Dawber, T. R. and McNamara, P. M. (1967). Relation of body weight to development of coronary heart disease. The Framingham study. *Circulation,* **35,** 734

100. Seltzer, C. C. (1966). Some re-evaluations of the body build and blood pressure study 1959, as related to the ponderal index, somatotype and mortality. *New Engl. J. Med.,* **274,** 254

101. Comstock, G. W., Kendrick, M. A. and Livesay, V. T. (1966). Subcutaneous fatness and mortality. *Amer. J. Epidemiol.,* **83,** 548

102. Anonymous (1969). Overweight and hypertension. *Nutr. Rev.*, **27,** 168

103. Reiniš, Z., Pokorný, J., Bazika, V., Heyrovský, A., Horáková, D., Klimešová A., Reisenauer, R., Maršíková, L., Kraus, H. and Klenka, L. (1974). Náklonnost k ischemické srdeční chorobe. *Čas. Lék. Čes.*, **113,** 116

104. Ošancová K. and Hejda, S. (1970). Nutrition and attitude to obesity. *Rev. Czechosl. Med.*, **16,** 131

4

The Experimental Psychology of Obesity

Orland W. Wooley and
Susan C. Wooley

Among the current theories purporting to explain the psychological basis of obesity in humans one of the earliest was that proposed by Hilde Bruch and summarised in her recent book[1] and among the first to generate experimental studies of the eating behaviour of the obese was Schachter's[2,3]. The central aetiological concepts of the two theories are similar. Bruch has proposed that eating disorders (obesity and anorexia nervosa) are caused by an inability to differentiate between bodily sensations and emotional states. Obese persons are viewed as having a faulty awareness of physiological hunger, so that emotional states are mislabelled as hunger; this leads to an excessive intake of food. Schachter's theory[2-4] consists of two hypotheses. The 'external hypothesis' states:

> . . . there is growing reason to suspect that the eating behavior of the obese is relatively unrelated to any internal gut state, but is, in large part, under external control; that is, eating behavior is initiated and terminated by stimuli external to the organism[2].

His 'internal hypothesis' states:

> The relationships are quite the reverse for the normal subject; his eating behavior seems directly linked to internal state but relatively unaffected by the external circumstances surrounding the eating routine and ritual[2].

In this chapter we first review the experimental evidence for these two hypotheses. Then follows a discussion of two more recent theoretical trends which can be viewed as extensions of the two original hypotheses. Finally, there will be a discussion of theoretical alternatives consistent with available evidence.

INTERNAL HYPOTHESIS

The concept 'internal state' (or 'internal cues') has most often been operationalised by manipulating caloric intake in the form of preloads or test meals. This manipulation has frequently been inadequate; subjects in some studies have known approximately how many calories they ingested and this knowledge could have had effects quite apart from the physiological effects of ingested calories. The only solution to the methodological problem of independently controlling calories and beliefs about calories is the use of liquid foods. The caloric density of liquid foods can be altered (while taste and other sensory cues are held constant) by differential use of artificial sweeteners and glucose (or sucrose), or by the addition of differing amounts of corn oil.

Studies designed to examine the effects of calorie content can be either short term or long term. Short-term studies investigate the effects of calories following a single meal or preload on such parameters as reported hunger, intake in a test meal, or appetite for food stimuli presented after ingestion of a meal or preload. Long-term studies investigate the effects of calories on daily caloric intake and body weight.

Short-term studies

Schachter's original hypothesis that non-obese people respond directly to internal cues was partially based on a study in which he found that non-obese subjects preloaded with roast beef sandwiches ate fewer crackers than those not preloaded; whereas preloaded obese subjects ate just as much as non-preloaded obese subjects[5].

Obviously, the preloaded non-obese subjects knew they had eaten the roast beef sandwiches, so an unequivocal conclusion about internal cues can not be drawn. Furthermore replication, or near replication, of this experiment have failed to yield similar results. Singh[6] reports: 'The fact that the deprivation condition did not significantly affect cracker consumption by either obese or normal subjects suggests that at least in this type of situation both normal and obese subjects ignore the "internal cues" associated with hunger.'

Price and Grinker[7] reported no significant difference between the number of crackers eaten in the preloaded and non-preloaded conditions for either the obese or the normal weight subjects.

Cabanac and Duclaux[8] found that non-obese, but not obese subjects liked the taste of sucrose samples of various concentrations (2.5 – 40%) less one hour after ingestion of 200 calories worth of glucose solution—an effect Cabanac[9] has labelled 'alliesthesia' (discussed in more detail below under 'Current Theories'). However, Wooley, Wooley, and Dunham[10] reported that a sweet but noncaloric cyclamate solution reduces liking for sucrose just as much as the caloric glucose solution in non-obese *and* obese subjects. The obese subjects in the latter study were college students who said they were not trying to lose weight at the time of the study. Cabanac and Duclaux' obese subjects were patients who wanted to lose weight. These subject differences may explain the lack of agreement with respect to obese-non-obese findings.

Meyer and Pudel[11] instructed overweight, underweight, and normal weight subjects to consume for breakfast and/or supper as much of a liquid food of fixed caloric density as they wanted over a period of ten days. Normal subjects consumed 80% of their meal in the first half of the 20 minute period allowed for meal consumption, while the obese subjects consumed only 50% of their meal in the first half of the period, i.e. approximately equal intake during each minute. The curve typical of the normals they call a 'biological satiation curve'; the curve typical of the obese they interpret 'as an expression of distorted perception of the degree of satiety'.

Spiegel[12] gave subjects of normal weight preloads which varied in caloric density from 0.25 kcal ml^{-1} to 1.8 kcal ml^{-1} but which were always the same volume for any given subject. For lunch, which in some cases was one hour and in other cases three to five hours after the preload, subjects drank as much Metrecal (1 kcal ml^{-1}) as they wanted. The volume of Metrecal ingested in the test meal did not vary as a function of the caloric density of the preload; nor did hunger or fullness ratings. The entire discussion section for this experiment reads: 'Experiment 1 clearly indicates that on liquid food, subjects do not compensate for changes in caloric intake within one meal or from one meal to the next by adjusting meal size.'

Jordan[13] in one of his earlier studies reported that subjects of normal weight did not increase the volume of self-regulated intragastric intake, or report increased hunger, when their Metrecal was, without their knowledge, diluted (nine parts water, one part Metrecal). In a more recent report[14], summarising a series of several experiments, Jordan concludes: 'Our preloading experiments showed that in short term experiments volume rather than calories is the most important variable.'

One of the few studies which manipulated simultaneously and independently both calories and those sensory qualities upon which beliefs about calories might reasonably be expected to be based was conducted by S. Wooley[15]. On four consecutive days, obese and non-obese subjects were given drinks (preloads) containing 200 or 600 calories (the difference made up by the addition of corn oil) and appearing half the time to be rich milkshakes and half the time to be low calorie diet liquids. Pilot research had confirmed that subjects thought the 'milkshakes' to be higher calorie than the 'diet liquids' but could not discriminate on the basis of taste between the high and low calorie version of each. Twenty minutes after consumption of the preload, a test meal of quarter sandwiches was presented. The major finding was that intake (number of quarter sandwiches eaten) varied as a function of the preload's sensory qualities, or (as post-experimental questioning revealed) beliefs about calories, but was unrelated to the actual number of calories in the preloads. This was true for the obese and the nonobese. The obese subjects did not eat more than the nonobese.

The studies discussed so far have failed to reveal any short term effects of caloric intake on subsequent feeding. Two possible explanations for this are: (1) not enough time had been allowed for calories to have an effect or (2) the conditions of the experiment did not maximise the

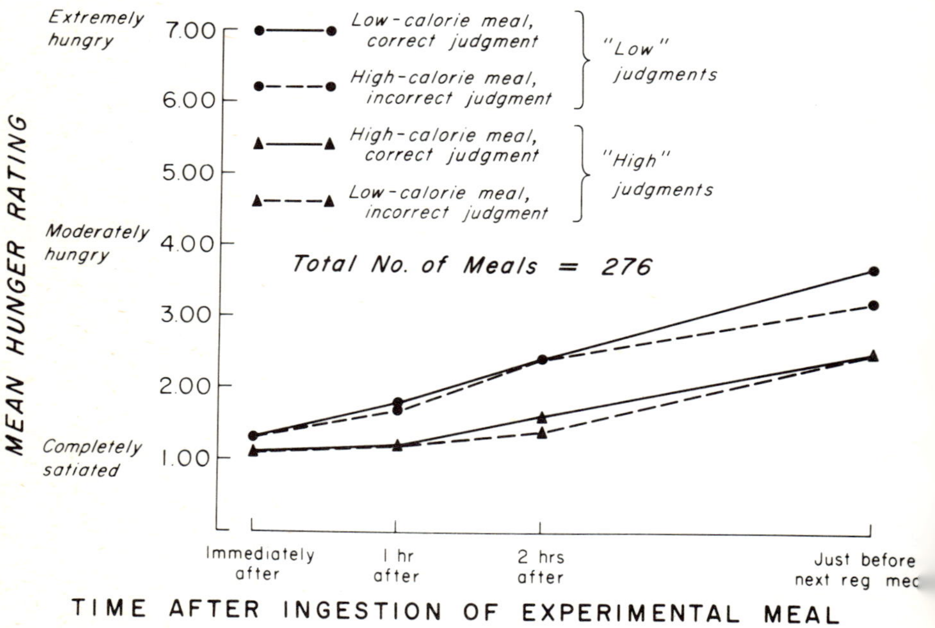

FIGURE 4.1 Mean hunger ratings of obese and non-obese subjects as a function of caloric content of the experimental meal, the correctness of the caloric judgement, and the time of the rating.

subjects' attentiveness to internal cues. O. Wooley, S. Wooley, and associates have attempted to determine if subjects can detect differences in hunger and satiety as a function of the caloric value of liquid meals when detection is made the main experimental task. Wooley, Wooley, and Dunham[16] gave obese and non-obese subjects high and low calorie liquid breakfasts or lunches. The two kinds of meal were always the same volume but differed in caloric density by a factor of two for any given subject. They could not be distinguished on the basis of taste, texture, or appearance. After each meal, subjects were asked to say whether they thought the meal was high calorie or low, and to report their hunger (7 point scale). Then, fifteen minutes, thirty minutes, one hour, two hours, just before and after the next meal, and just before the next experimental meal (the next day) they again guessed high or low and reported their hunger. Neither the guesses nor the hunger ratings were at all related to the actual caloric density of the liquid meal. This was true of both the obese and non-obese subjects. They could not correctly guess at any time during the twenty-four hours between experimental meals whether a meal was high calorie or low. Furthermore, their hunger ratings were highly inversely related to their initial guess (i.e. greater hunger if the first guess was low). Figure 4.1 presents hunger ratings following high and low calorie meals as a function of actual and believed caloric density in a replication[7] of the original study. (The replication study used a larger number of subjects and was run under more tightly controlled experimental conditions; the major results were the same in every respect.)

In sum, in studies where the concept 'internal cues' has been operationalised by a systematic manipulation of caloric density of ingested food, and where food intake or perceived hunger have served as dependent variables, there is almost no unequivocal experimental evidence to support the hypothesis that humans, even those of normal body weight, are sensitive to short term internal cues of satiety. (Furthermore, other studies[18,19] have shown little relationship between reported hunger and gastric contractions, which Schachter specifically mentions as a possible 'internal cue'.) On the other hand some of these same studies[15-17] have shown that what a person believes about the satiating effect of ingested food is a powerful determinant of short term intake, and of hunger following intake. These demonstrations of the influence of cognitive factors on intake and reported hunger are at variance with changes in insulin, blood sugar and hypothalamic activity known to occur when food is ingested.

Taking a different approach, Wooley, Wooley and Woods[20] investigated the effect of calories, ingested in the form of high and low calorie liquid lunches (900 calories and 450 calories, respectively, but of equal volume, 900 cc), on appetite, one hour later, for a highly palatable food stimulus, (either cholocate cake à la mode or a fish sandwich). As a possible involuntary measure of appetite, salivation was used. They found that with the non-obese subjects the food stimulus elicited a salivary response well above the baseline salivation level (measured with no food present) on low calorie days, but not on high calorie days. Food appeal ratings by these same (non-obese) subjects of how 'appetising' the food stimulus looked just prior to its consumption, were significantly lower on high calorie days than on low calorie days. With the obese subjects the food stimulus elicited a salivary response above baseline on both high and low calorie days; however, the mean salivary response on low calorie days was significantly greater than that on high calorie days. Food appeal ratings by the obese subjects were unaffected by calories. Hunger ratings made one hour after the liquid lunches were unrelated to calories in both the obese and non-obese. (Post-experimental questioning showed that the subjects were unable as a group to guess correctly which of the meals were high and which low calorie; and that there was no relationship between the guesses and the salivary responses to the food stimulus.) Apparently, appetite was almost completely inhibited in the non-obese by the high calorie meal, but only partially so in the obese.

With reference to the original question of sensitivity to internal cues, these results show that obese subjects *are* sensitive to calories; their response to a palatable food *is* affected by recent caloric intake. The fact that this response is only partially inhibited by doubling the caloric intake calls to mind Singh's[6] response inhibition deficit theory (discussed below). However, equally plausible would be an interpretation which held that the appetitive response to highly palatable food by obese subjects was so strong that a greater caloric intake was required to inhibit it, i.e. a case of greater excitation rather than lesser inhibition. Such an interpretation emphasises the potential role of palatability in evoking appetitive responses. The concept of palatability is, as yet, poorly defined and studied in the experimental literature. In the animal literature it is manipulated by adulterating food with quinine or other unpalatable adulterants or enriching it with fats or sweetening agents. However, even though some investigators[21-23] have used such methods with humans, it would appear that a more sophisticated approach is required in the study of human eating behaviour; especially in the light of the apparent discontinuity between the physiological response to food (as indexed by salivation) and the cognitive response to it (as measured by hunger ratings).

Long-term studies

Wooley[24] instructed hospitalised obese and non-obese subjects (none of whom were patients) to drink nothing but liquid food *ad lib.* for five baseline and ten experimental days. For five of the experimental days the liquid food was high calorie; for the other five days it was low calorie; the two kinds of food tasted alike. Subjects drank a greater *volume* of liquid food during the low calorie period (mean of 2374 ml *v.* 2091 ml during the high period), but their *caloric* intake was greater during the high calorie period (mean of 3066 calories/day *v.* 1920 calories/day during the low calorie period). Post-experimental questioning revealed no evidence that the subjects were aware of the change in caloric density. There were no obese - non-obese differences in intake, but the obese subjects' reported hunger (rated every four hours throughout the day) increased significantly as the experiment progressed.

Campbell *et al.*[25] report that their five hospitalised non-obese subjects on an all-liquid food regimen adjusted promptly to concealed changes in caloric density of the liquid food and maintained body weight. Their four obese subjects (who were patients who presumably wanted to lose weight) did not ingest enough of the liquid food to maintain their weight and did not change their intake in response to changes in caloric density of the liquid food. Their two juvenile obese subjects drank large amounts of the liquid food, but only one adjusted to changes in caloric density.

Speigel[12] studied non-hospitalised non-obese subjects who ate nothing but liquid food for ten to twenty-one days during which time the caloric density was switched at least once for each subject without his being told. On the basis of her results she was able to classify six of the fifteen subjects as regulators, six as non-regulators, and three as 'questionable'. The six regulators showed an 88% compensation in two to five days for diet dilution by eating more (i.e. increasing the volume of their intake) and maintaining a stable weight. The mean caloric intake of the non-regulators on the diluted diet was 40-59% of the undiluted diet, and they lost weight. The questionable subjects did not compensate for the diet dilution, but neither did they lose weight.

In summary, although the number of subjects actually studied is small, it appears that some people are capable of responding by appropriately altering their calorie intake to caloric dilutions and enrichments of their all-liquid diet, even though they are unaware of the changes in caloric density. However, the response seems sluggish and imprecise in all but five non-obese subjects of Campbell *et al.*[25] The available data offers few clues as to what factors might account for these individual differences. Very long term studies which relate daily caloric intake to changes in amount of stored body fat are needed, especially with the increase in the popularity of ponderostat-type theories (discussed below).

EXTERNAL HYPOTHESIS

There is, of course, no doubt that food intake is affected by environmental factors. The hypothesis proposed by Schachter and his colleagues is that the intake of the obese is *more* affected by external stimuli than that of normals. Studies which demonstrate a failure of the obese to show decreases in food intake comparable with those of normals following pre-loading do not necessarily bear on this hypothesis. That is, failure to curtail intake does not imply external control, just as successful limitation of intake does not imply internal control. Studies relevant to the external hypothesis are those in which external stimuli are manipulated and the magnitude of responses of obese and normal subjects to the manipulation are compared.

Palatability

The largest group of such studies involve manipulations of palatability of food. In the earliest study, Nisbett[21] predicted that obese subjects would eat less bad tasting ice cream and more good tasting ice cream than normals. The hypothesis was not confirmed; rather, the obese ate more of both kinds of ice cream. However, *post hoc* ratings of liking showed a stronger relationship to intake in the obese at the high end of the rated palatability dimension. Obese and normal subjects ate similar amounts of ice cream if they rated it poor, but the obese ate more ice cream than normals if they rated it very good. Similarly, Price and Grinker[7] found that in a cracker tasting experiment, obese subjects ate more well-liked crackers than normals, but the same amount of disliked crackers. Schachter has reported the results of an (unpublished) study by Decke[22] which is the only study showing obese-normal differences at both ends of the palatability spectrum. Decke found that the obese ate more good milkshake but less bad milkshake than normals. Jackson[23] studied intake of sandwiches rated 'very good' and 'very bad' and found no differences in intake of good and bad sandwiches by either obese or normal subjects, despite complaints by subjects about the bad sandwiches. This points to the possibility that demand characteristics represent a particular problem in short-term laboratory studies. This problem is discussed by Price and Grinker[7] with special reference to brief exposure studies involving deception, and by Bauer[26] who stresses the possible effects of shame over obesity on experimental results.

The problem of subject compliance with demand characteristics is probably not so prominent in long-term studies. Several comparisons have been made of the intake of obese and normal subjects of an *ad lib.* liquid diet over a period of weeks. Schachter has suggested that because liquid diet foods are bland and uninteresting they are particularly appropriate for demonstrating the differential responsiveness of obese and normals to external factors. Hashim and Van Itallie[27] reported that obese subjects hospitalised for weight loss ate far less liquid diet than normal volunteers, and many fewer calories per day than when eating standard hospital diet. However, O. Wooley[24] found no differences in the amounts of liquid food consumed by obese and non-obese inmates over a 15-day period. Differences between these two studies include the motivation of subjects to lose weight and the setting in which eating took place. In Hashim and Van Itallie's study food was dispensed by a machine in an isolated location; in Wooley's study inmates could eat together, permitting social facilitation (which was considered as an 'external cue' by Schachter but which is obviously separable from palatability).

In a recent naturalistic study of the effect of palatability on intake, Wooley *et al.*[28] observed 2500 meal choices of patrons rated obese or normal at two cafeterias representing distinctly different levels of

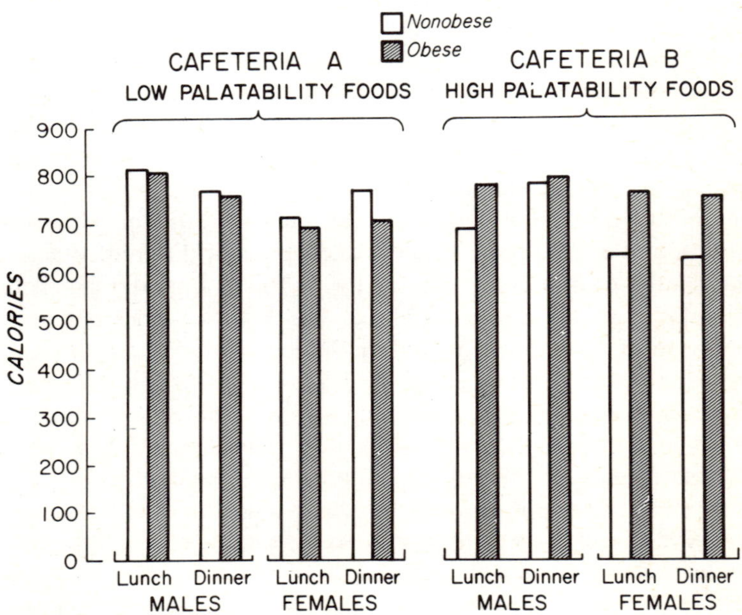

FIGURE 4.2 Caloric value of meals (N = 2500) selected by cafeteria patrons as a function of estimated weight, sex, and palatability of food.

palatability. One was an employees cafeteria serving mediocre institutional food; the other a fancy suburban cafeteria serving a large variety of palatable foods, attractively displayed. The caloric value of meal choices as a function of weight, meal (lunch or dinner), and location are shown in Figure 4.2. The obese ate an average of 18 calories less than the normals at the plain cafeteria, and a mean 100 calories more per meal at the fancy cafeteria.

This finding is consistent with other studies reviewed in showing that the obese appear to be somewhat hyper-responsive to palatability, but only at high levels of palatability. That is, the obese tend to eat somewhat more than normals when the food is very good. The evidence that low palatability leads to under-eating in the obese is unconvincing at this time.

A distinction should be made between the effects on intake of palatable stimuli in the immediate environment and a tendency to seek out opportunities to eat palatable food. Goldman *et al.*[29] reported that obese college students were more likely to cancel dormitory food contracts in order to eat in better restaurants. This constitutes a different phenomenon and is a result difficult to reconcile with Nisbett's[30] finding that obese subjects tend to eat as many sandwiches as are placed on a table before them, being unwilling to cross the room to obtain more. One interpretation proposed by Nisbett was an unwillingness of the obese to work for food. It is possible that this was an experiment in which reticence of the obese to eat more than the suggested norm (as noted by Bauer[26]) represents a particularly difficult methodological problem.

The study of cafeteria meal selections contained some data consistent with the findings of Goldman *et al.*[29] The magnitude of the effect of palatability on intake was the same at lunch and dinner. However, the proportion of obese eating in the two locations at different times varied significantly. At dinner as compared with lunch, a greater proportion of the sample at the fancy cafeteria was obese, whereas a smaller proportion of the sample at the employees cafeteria was obese. Since most people have more freedom of choice in selecting a location to eat dinner, these data suggest, in keeping with the results of Goldman *et al.*, that given a choice the obese seek out better food. Thus the direct influence of palatability on intake and the tendency to seek out good food appear to be additive effects. Obese—normal differences in food seeking or 'cue management' would serve to enhance the importance of the effects of palatability on intake.

Although most studies of palatability have examined the relationship between presence of palatable food stimuli and resultant intake, there is another interesting issue: the delayed effects of ingestion of low

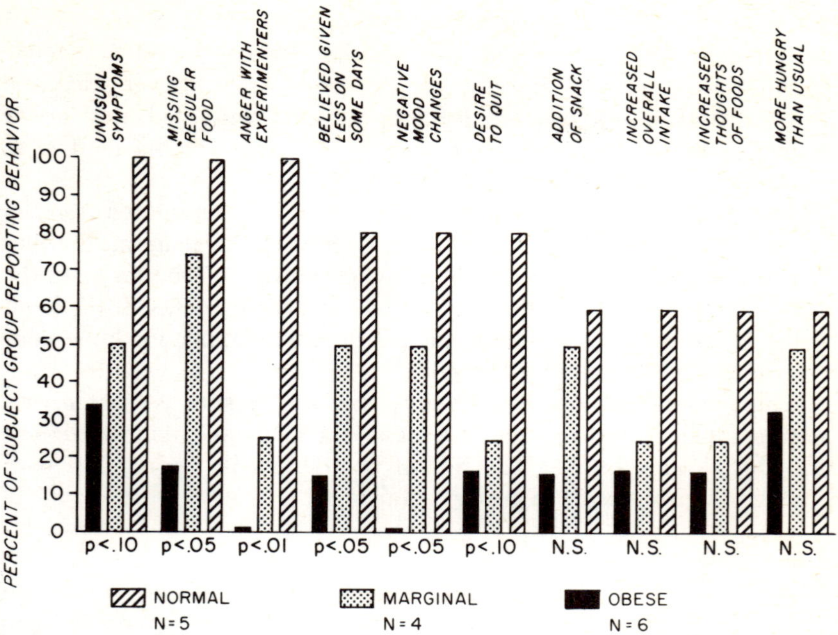

FIGURE 4.3 Reports of subjects, grouped by weight, on the effects of replacement of one meal a day with a liquid meal for three weeks. Information obtained from post-experimental interviews.

palatability meals. O. Wooley[24] found that hunger ratings of obese inmates eating an *ad lib.* liquid diet increased steadily over days, suggesting that they interpreted the desire for something besides liquid food as hunger. Wooley (unpublished data) interviewed all the subjects who had participated in an experiment requiring the replacement of one ordinary meal a day for several weeks with a liquid meal ranging from 30% below to 30% above the individual's usual caloric intake. Figure 4.3 shows the distribution of reported reactions of obese, marginally obese, and normal subjects. The responses did not appear to relate to caloric value of the meals, but rather tended to occur consistently or not at all in each individual. The obese tolerated the minor deprivation with considerably less reported discomfort and fewer instances of compensatory supplemental food intake, a finding which may be attributable to their prior experience with liquid diet foods or other weight reduction programs, or to a reluctance to complain, or admit to additional eating. The responses of the obese cannot be related to Schachter's external hypothesis because the extent to which the subjects were exposed to food stimuli following ingestion of the liquid meal is unknown. However, the responses of the normal subjects whose nutritional needs were met is inconsistent with: Schachter's hypothesis. Jordan[13] obtained similar findings in studies of normal subjects with oral, intragastric, and simultaneous oral-intragastric feeding. Subjects consumed most in the latter condition, suggesting that sensory experience of the food is an important component of satiety.

In another recent study, Wooley *et al.*[31] manipulated sensory satisfaction by requiring subjects to eat precisely the same meal either hurriedly or slowly with instructions to concentrate on the taste. In the condition designed to produce enhanced sensory experience of the food, subjects salivated less while viewing a different palatable food one hour later than when required to eat quickly.

Thus, palatability or, more broadly, sensory pleasure associated with eating appears to affect both the intake of foods and the duration of satiety following intake. The role of palatability in the regulation of intake will be discussed in greater detail later.

Cue saliency

The second external factor studied in some detail is saliency of external food-related cues. Goldman *et al.*[29] found that during Yom Kippur fasts, the obese showed a greater differential in retroactive ratings of unpleasantness of the fast as a function of where they spent their time (home *v.* synagogue) than did normal subjects. Schachter described a study by Ross[32] showing that degree of illumination of a bowl of cashews affected the intake of the obese but not that of the non-obese. The effect of heightened cue prominence was, however, rather small, increasing the intake of cashews by the obese by only some 18 g.

Levitz[33] has reviewed studies varying visibility of food. Johnson[34] showed that obese subjects would not work as hard as normals to obtain sandwiches which were wrapped as opposed to ones which were readily visible. However, several other studies[35,36] comparing intakes of liquid food from visible and nonvisible sources suggest that both normal and obese subjects eat *less* when food is visible. Since it could be argued that the sight of liquid food is not as potent a stimulus as the sight of more palatable foods and that an important variable in these studies may be the ease of monitoring intake, these studies require cautious interpretation. However, Levitz[33] reports results of an experiment by Stunkard and Levitz[37] giving strong support to the counter-hypothesis that cue saliency affects obese and normal subjects equally. He observed 3265 dessert selections of cafeteria patrons rated normal and obese. Following baseline, low calorie desserts were placed in a forward position on dessert racks, and high calorie ones far in the rear. Later, these positions were reversed. Normal subjects were highly susceptible to both manipulations. Obese subjects increased their selection of low calorie desserts when they were prominently displayed, but did not respond to availability of high calorie desserts, suggesting a resistance to external cues presumably based on voluntary controls. Similarly, closing the lid on the ice cream freezer resulted in an approximately 70% reduction in ice cream selections for both normal and obese subjects.

On the basis of current evidence it cannot be concluded that cue saliency affects normals and obese differently. Only two studies involving observation of intake have confirmed this phenomenon, while several others, inluding one involving large numbers of subjects in a non-experimental setting, have not.

Clock time

A third factor hypothesised to have exaggerated affects on intake of the obese is clock time. Goldman *et al.*[29] reported that obese flight personnel reported less discomfort from disruption of eating habits due to time zone changes, than did normal weight ones. The only other directly relevant evidence is Schachter and Gross'[38] finding that the obese increase their intake when led to believe by a rigged clock that it is dinner time. However, this manipulation also affected normals who curtailed their intake, probably, according to the authors, so as not to spoil their dinner. Schachter and Gross' additional finding that the obese eat more irregularly than normals over the weekends when social cues to eat are less prominent also tends to argue against clock time *per se* as a critical variable.

Social and cognitive cues

Finally, there are a host of social and cognitive cues known to affect eating. Originally included in the definition of external cues, Nisbett and Storms[39] have suggested they should be removed from that category, since they seem to affect normals as much, if not more, than the obese. These include belief about caloric value[15,39], intake by an experimental shill[39], and the size of food units presented, all of which may carry certain social cues about expected intake as well as differentially affecting cognitive monitoring[15,36,39].

We may conclude that the external hypothesis of food intake has received substantial validation as a predictor of obese-normal differences only with respect to palatability. Having narrowed the range of relevant cues, 'external' may no longer seem an apt label, since sensory cues may readily be conceived as playing a role in other kinds of processes; for example, conditioning. This issue will be discussed in greater detail later.

CURRENT THEORIES

Thus far only evidence relevant to Schachter's original hypotheses has been considered. There are however at least two other trends in current theorising which go beyond Schachter's views. One is mainly social-psychological, the other is physiological. The social-psychological theoretical efforts generalise the external hypothesis to include *all* environmental stimuli, not just food-related ones. The physiological theories focus on the effects of weight reduction.

Social-psychological extension of the external hypothesis

The social-psychological theory holds that obese people are overly responsive to all stimuli, not just food or food-related stimuli[40]. Rodin[41] and Pliner[42,43] have contributed most of the experimental evidence in support of this viewpoint. Rodin, characterising the eating behaviour of the obese as 'stimulus bound', and predicting that 'they should be more responsive to any prominent stimulus', found that overweight subjects were more distracted than non-obese by interesting tape recordings. (These tapes instructed subjects to: 'Picture people whose faces were wholly burned, their eyesockets hollow, the fluid from their melted eyes running down their cheeks', or 'Consider how the impact of your (leukaemia) would . . . affect your every significant relationship . . . who would feel distressed and who would be put upon . . . who would be glad to see you dying in great pain and suffering'.) Likening obese people to rats with ventromedial hypothalamic lesions, she concludes, 'overweight people are highly reactive to compelling emotional stimuli, i.e. the tapes. The obese appear to be stimulus bound for emotionality as well as for eating, thinking, and attention. It is tempting to consider the engaging predictions which can be derived, without too much fancy footwork from these findings. On the whole, obese individuals whose thinking seems to be stimulus bound should be less creative than normals. On the other hand, they should be marvellous accountants, at least when undistracted.

During the last three days of their experiment, Meyer and Pudel[11] applied 'stressors' (monotonous sound, irregular noise, and an insoluble puzzle) while their subjects ate liquid meals. They report 'a clear tendency towards hyperphagia in the obese group. The underweight subjects tend to react hypophagically'. If these stressors are seen as distracting stimuli, the results (hyperphagia in the obese) would appear to be in contradiction to Rodin's[41] finding that the obese are more likely than the non-obese to be distracted by extraneous stimuli away from an ongoing task. However, Meyer and Pudel's procedure is not described fully enough to determine whether it is comparable with Rodin's.

Pliner[42] found that obese subjects overestimated the duration of a tape recording of 'beeps' (0.2-second tone pulses of frequency 500 cylces/second) if the beeps were 90 decibels ('high-salience') and underestimated if they were 45 decibels ('low-salience'). She also found[43] that obese subjects reported they spent more time thinking about a scene (mountain or beach) if a slide of the scene was present. She discusses a qualification of the externality hypothesis : 'It is only to stimuli high in salience that the obese are more responsive than normals; they are actually less responsive to stimuli low in salience[42].' Since her subjects did not report the 90 decibel beeps more 'annoying' than the 45 decibel ones, she concludes (in apparent disagreement with Rodin): 'It appears unlikely that time estimation results . . . could be alternatively interpreted in terms of emotionality rather than salience[42].'

Singh[6] and his co-workers[44] have proposed the hypothesis that obese persons are deficient in inhibitory responses—*any* responses, not just eating responses. Singh[6] found that obese subjects did not eat more (in fact, they ate less) than normals, even though the food stimuli (crackers) were prominently displayed (salient) if the response required to obtain the food was incompatible with an earlier learned response. Subjects were trained on a piece of apparatus which 'consisted of a 32-gauge stainless steel wire 36 inches long which was twisted into inverted U bends and attached to a wooden stand. The wire contained 25 crackers . . . and 15 metal discs. Both crackers and metal discs had a hole in the centre and could be easily moved along the bent wire and removed'[6].

During testing 'subjects in the incompatible condition moved the crackers in the direction opposite to training, while subjects in the compatible condition moved the crackers in the same direction as in training'. The crackers were eaten after being removed.

Generalising to non-eating responses, Singh[6] found that obese subjects, given interfering pre-training prior to a time estimation task, do less well than non-obese subjects on the task. He also found that obese subjects showed a greater Einstellung effect ('inferred when subjects persist in using some initial method of solving problems in spite of the fact that other methods, some of which are much simpler and more direct than the initial method, are feasible', p. 231). He states: 'Thus, it may be concluded that obese subjects compared to normals show a greater resistance to change habits (sic), whether motoric or mental.' Overeating, in his system, is due to a 'deficit in terminating the response of eating'. He speculated that an inability to suppress negative emotional reactions to bad tasting and positive ones to good tasting food might explain the sometimes reported finickiness of obese people. (The phenomenon of finickiness is not clearly documented in humans as noted in the section on the External Hypothesis.) When work is required to obtain food, perhaps a negative emotional response is evoked (drive frustration?) which obese subjects have difficulty suppressing, so they eat less. According to this view, obese subjects are not more responsive to emotional stimuli, they are just less capable of suppressing emotional responses.

Singh *et al.*[44] report some further results which they interpret in accordance with the response inhibition deficit theory. Obese subjects took longer and made more errors on a hand-eye co-ordination task when required to use their non-preferred hand. The theory was not confirmed by an experiment which involved a discriminative reaction-time test; when the S+ (response required) and the S— (withholding of response required) were reversed, the obese subjects responded faster than normals and did not make significantly more errors.

Physiological theories

Cabanac[9] and his associates[45] have proposed a 'ponderostat' theory which is an elaboration of Schachter's internal hypothesis. According to the ponderostat theory, the taste of food becomes less pleasant following ingestion of sufficient calories to satisfy the body's need for food, and cessation of eating is the result (the process is called 'alliesthaesia'), but only if the individual is at his ponderostat or regulated weight. All physiological and behavioural controls work to maintain or defend the ponderostat weight, which may be average, below average, or well above average for any given individual. When a person whose actual body weight is below his ponderostat weight (and most obese people are seen as fitting this description), the taste of food is unaffected by ingestion of calories, and remains so until the weight difference is eliminated. In effect, this theory says Schachter's internal hypothesis holds only for people who are at their regulated weight; only at that weight is there sensitivity to internal cues.

Some of the evidence for 'alliesthaesia', a central concept in the ponderostat theory was presented earlier[8,9]. Independent evidence incompatible with Cabanac's interpretation of his data was also presented[10]. Elsewhere Cabanac, Duclaux, and Spector[45] reported a reduction of the alliesthaesia effect with a voluntary 10% weight loss and a return of alliesthaesia upon regaining the weight. (This finding is weakened by the fact that the three subjects were the experimenters themselves; they were necessarily aware of which responses would confirm or disconfirm their hypothesis.) Using Cabanac's own procedures, Grinker and Hirsch[46] reported that their reduced obese subjects showed as powerful an alliesthaesia effect as non-obese subjects. Before weight reduction these subjects did not show alliesthaesia. These findings are both in disagreement with the ponderostat theory. Cabanac's alliesthaesia concept represents an attempt to demonstrate a relationship between weight loss or gain (below or above the pre-set weight) and a short-term intake variable (preference for sweet taste). The failure to do so lends credence to Price and Grinker's[7] warning: 'The slowness of caloric adjustment and the high degree of variability in short term experiments point to the dangers of basing a theory of long term eating behaviour on results obtained from brief-exposure tests.'

Results which are supportive of one implication of the ponderostat theory (i.e. obese persons respond 'normally' to food deprivation severe enough to cause them to drop below their regulated body weight) is provided by Glucksman, Hirsch, Grinker, and associates[47-50]. Patients who were obese as children (juvenile obese whose regulated body weight is high) respond in much the same way as non-obese people do when starved:

> Perhaps the most intriguing aspect of this study was that the removal of obesity by means of caloric deprivation led to behavioral alterations similar to those observed in the starvation of non-obese individuals. That is, there was evidence of hunger symptoms, hostility-aggression, fantasies and dreams of food or eating, diet-breaking, anxiety, and depressive symptoms. Concurrent with these behavioral changes were morphologic and biochemical alterations of adipose tissue indistinguishable from those found in the adipose tissue of starved non-obese individuals. It is entirely possible that weight reduction, instead of resulting in a normal state for obese patients, results in an abnormal state resembling that of starved non-obese individuals[49].

Patients whose obesity is adult onset suffer no such effects[50].

These investigators also report[46] that after weight reduction juvenile onset obese subjects underestimated the duration of one second and three second time intervals. They interpret this as a slowing of the 'internal clock', reflecting a slowing of metabolism. Grinker and Hirsch[46] state:

> The alterations in timing perception and the correlated changes in effect might well be an expression of the biological consequences of

> weight reduction. The response of the juvenile-onset obese subject may represent a pattern of energy conservation aimed at maintaining homeostasis of fat storage. The absence of these changes in adult-onset subjects again suggests that age of onset is an important variable in describing the nature of obesity[46] (p. 355).

(See Nisbett[51] for a review which attempts to synthesise the human and animal work in this area. Hervey[52] has suggested that a hormonal-hypothalamic lipostatic system may exist (see Chapter 1). Jordan[53] discusses the evidence for the ponderostat concept and its implications for treatment of obesity (see Chapter 6).)

THEORETICAL ALTERNATIVES

Feeding behaviour has been conceptualised as governed by long-term and short-term regulatory processes. The variable of most interest in long-term regulation is body weight, or amount of body fat. Theories which attempt to explain this process are called ponderostat[9,45] or lipostat[52] theories. The variables of most interest in short-term regulation are meal size (the problem of satiety or cessation of eating) and meal-to-meal interval (the problem of hunger or initiation of eating).

Sclafani and Kluge[54] have recently presented and tested (on rats) a lipostat theory. They state:

> The dual lipostat model proposed here obviously is an incomplete model of feeding and body weight regulation. It emphasizes long-term regulation, and although it has been related to meal size, the model offers little concerning the short-term control of food intake.

The same problems pertain to Cabanac's ponderostat theory despite his attempt to relate weight regulation to short term intake. The alliesthaesia hypothesis proposes that once the body's needs for energy are met, the taste of the food being ingested changes from palatable to unpalatable. However in most meal situations eating stops long before the ingested food is absorbed, i.e. before the energy needs can be replenished. In fact, a change in preference for sucrose—which Cabanac has interpreted as evidence of alliesthaesia—may occur even when *no* energy needs are met[10].

The fact that eating stops before bodily needs are met, (or that when it stops does not depend upon the caloric content of what is being ingested), has been of particular interest to those experimental psychologists who study learning. The two major theories of learning

(Pavlovian and operant conditioning) are based largely on observation of the effects on behaviour of systematic manipulation of food and food-related variables. Food has been for both the most thoroughly studied 'reinforcement'. The general problem of reinforcement for the physiological psychologist is stated by Valenstien[55]:

> There now exists considerable evidence that the reinforcement process does not always depend upon 'feedback' from physiological consequences of the behaviour. Sweet substances are ingested and bitter substances are rejected before their ultimate beneficial or harmful consequences can be sensed. What is required is some mechanism to bridge the gap between behavior and the biological consequences of the behavior.

Considering the importance of food in the history of learning theory, it is striking that only recently have the concepts of learning been focused on eating behaviour itself. There are two theoretical papers[56,57] each of which uses the concepts of one of the two conditioning theories to explain how sensory properties of food (e.g. taste) could become, through a process of conditioning, the stimulus (either a conditioned stimulus, CS, of Pavlovian theory, or a discriminative stimulus, SD, of operant theory) and how the physiological, nutritional and metabolic effects of ingested food could be the reinforcement (either the unconditioned stimulus, UCS, of Pavlovian theory, or the reinforcing stimulus of operant theory). The major obstacle to this idea has always been the long delay between the ingestion of food and the eventual physiological effects. Both the theoretical papers quoted focus on this point; both deal principally with learned aversions to foods with negative physiological consequences.

Rozin and Kalat[56] point out that rats learn an aversion to diets associated with thiamine deficiency—an aversion which persists even after the deficiency has been eliminated. They say:

> We can consider the deficient diet as a CS and the nausea or other ill effects produced by its ingestion as a UCS. Presumably, the classically conditioned 'ill effects' lead to avoidance of the familiar food.

The long-delay problem is handled by a concept of 'belongingness':

> Belongingness is the tendency to associate tastes with aversive internal consequences as opposed to associating either elements with anything else . . . Gastrointestional and related internal events are . . . very likely to be initiated or influenced by substances eaten,

> and taste receptors, by virtue of their location, provide information about these same substances.

Revusky and Garcia[57] attempt to use operant learning principles to explain aversions to saccharin solutions which develop if its ingestion is followed (up to six hours later) by poison or X-radiation. They handle the long delay problem in much the same way Rozin and Kalat did:

> . . . the fact that infra-humans . . . can associate over long delays strongly suggests that there is an innate selective association of flavors with physiological aftereffects.

They invoke the concept of 'stimulus relevance':

> The relevance principle responsible for association of delayed physiological aftereffects with flavors is that a flavor has high associative strength relative to a physiological consequence, while an exteroceptive stimulus has low associative strength.

And later:

> Since rats are likely to consume a number of substances prior to toxicosis, how can they detect which of the substances actually produced the toxicosis? . . . The logical solution is for the rat not to associate familiar, relevant stimuli with a novel toxicosis, if novel, relevant stimuli also occur.

LeMagnen[58] has also developed a theory in which food flavours, through a process of conditioning, come to influence intake in a regulatory manner. However, instead of negative consequences such as toxicosis or nausea, he has manipulated the *caloric-nutritive consequences* associated with different flavours. He found, for example, that if ingestion of a food flavoured with flavour A was always followed by an intravenous injection of glucose, and if ingestion of the same food flavoured with flavour B was followed by an injection of saline, voluntary intake of the A-flavoured food, but not that of the B-flavoured food, gradually decreased. In the long run (over a period of two to three weeks) relative intake of the two flavours worked to equalise their caloric consequences. This differential intake of the two flavours continued for up to six days after the injections were discontinued. So, apparently, when the caloric-metabolic consequences associated with a given flavour repeatedly over-satiate the animal—when these consequences are more than required for 'regulation'—a relative aversion for that flavour develops.

What has been dealt with so far is the problem of satiety, the question of why eating stops. Some justification has been found in the animal literature for viewing this aspect of eating behaviour as governed by specialised laws of learning. How useful this view will be in understanding human eating behaviour or obesity remains to be seen.

What has not been dealt with is the problem of hunger, the question of why eating starts. Lepkovsky[59] has written:

> Accumulative evidence suggests that the urge to eat is a primitive, *unconditioned* instinct that exists at all times in all animals whether or not they possess an alimentary system. In other words, hunger exists at all time unless inhibited . . . Presumably (in higher animals), the lateral hypothalamus stimulates hunger at all times unless it is inhibited by the ventromedial nucleus (our italics).

How well do these concepts explain the major conclusions of the review section of this paper? In studies[13,14] of single meals in which sensory qualities were held constant and caloric density varied, intake was not related to calories. Le Magnen[60] has written,

> In this learning process, the systematically active nutritional properties of the food act as . . . 'reinforcers' of the adapted appetite while the short-tem control of this feeding response [is] entirely dependent on the sensory action of the same food.

It follows that if sensory properties of two foods are the same, the 'feeding response' to the foods should be the same. Similarly, manipulation of caloric density of preloads[12,15-17] matched for taste did not affect later intake or reported hunger. In some instances[6,7], even when caloric pre-loading was undisguised, pre-loads had no effect on later intake, a finding which seems to suggest that within a single meal the sensory properties of the food may be so important a determinant of quantity consumed that it can override the effects of a variety of prior manipulations.

Another major conclusion was that long term response to disguised switches in the caloric density of liquid foods was sluggish and imprecise. Again this is in agreement with Le Magnen's[58] finding that differential intake of two flavours which had been associated with different internal consequences lasted up to six days after the caloric consequences had been equalised.

Another conclusion is that the obese are somewhat hyper-responsive to palatability factors. Although most studies have shown the intake of both normal and obese subjects to be related to preference ratings or manipulated palatability, the effect is slightly stronger in the obese. One explanation of this obese - non-obese difference starts with an assumption made by ponderostat theorists[9,51], who assume that because the obese are below their regulated weight, they are physiologically hungrier than usual. (Note, however, Nisbett's[51] statement: 'The present view that the obese may be below their set points has received no direct test as of the present time, and is in fact the weakest link in the present theoretical position.') If the obese are hungrier more often than normals then they will eat under high deprivation conditions more often than normals. In answer to the question of whether there are learned preferences, as well as learned aversions, Rozin and Kalat[56] state:

> Revusky . . . performed a series of experiments to demonstrate that food with clear positive consequences would be preferred to foods with relatively neutral consequences. In his simple design, rats were fed one nutrient solution while hungry and a different one when satiated. After five days of this training, a significant preference developed in a two-bottle test for the solution drunk while deprived. This result is interpreted in terms of the greater (delayed) reinforcing effect of the solution drunk during deprivation.

Such a process might explain the development of strong preferences in the obese which in turn may lead to increased intake of preferred foods, or to an increased probability that eating will be initiated when the preferred foods are available, or both. Le Magnen[60] states:

> Positive palatability acts like hunger. The oral sensory properties of food act to facilitate differential eating as does internal depletion or hunger. These two factors (internal and peripheral) are additive in the initiation of feeding.

He presents as confirming evidence the finding that the 'endogramme' characteristics normally associated with hunger (rapidity, intensity, and amount of chewing for each unit of food eaten), recorded as subjects ate eight different foods of varying palatability, correlated positively with amount eaten of the different foods. Jacobs and Sharma[61] have demonstrated that hungry animals (dogs and rats) are more responsive to palatability factors than non-hungry ones, a finding consistent with Le Magnen's[60] statement that hunger and palatability are additive.

So, these concepts borrowed from the animal literature seem to explain some of the more general conclusions drawn from the review of the human studies. However, before these concepts can be applied in new experiments with humans, some means of measuring hunger (i.e. 'urge to eat', 'lateral hypothalamic' activity, *physiological* hunger) in humans is needed.

The study of hunger in humans poses many problems. Hunger ratings have certain drawbacks, some empirical, some rational. For example, length of deprivation should affect hunger (as described by Lepkovsky[59]) simply as a result of dissipation of inhibition over time. However, it is impossible to vary length of time since the last meal without human subjects having some idea of how long ago that meal occurred. This knowledge contaminates hunger ratings; it is impossible to know the relative contributions of length of deprivation *per se* and knowledge of length of deprivation to the observed variance in hunger ratings. When relative deprivation was manipulated without the subject's knowledge, as with high and low calorie meals[12,16,17,20] hunger ratings were not found to be a function of this difference in caloric content of the preload. Nevertheless hunger ratings have been shown to correlate highly with food eaten at a subsequent meal; this has been taken to support the view that hunger ratings can reflect 'the desire for food'[62]. Furthermore hunger rating scales of the linear analogue type can discriminate effectively between different doses of anorectic drugs (see Chapter 7).

When using such measures we should remember that reports of hunger are subject to consistent response biases as Stunkard and Koch[63,64] have shown. Furthermore hunger ratings are potentially vague; little attempt has been made (or described) to control what the subject is thinking about when the rating is made. If his attention is on some specific food (acutally present or imagined) which he likes or dislikes his hunger rating may be altered towards increased or decreased hunger as compared with a situation where his attention is not on food.

If hunger ratings are insufficient to study the urge to eat in humans, and, obviously, the methods of the rat lab are unsuitable, what alternative exists? Tietelbaum[65] has written:

> Lateral hypothalamic activity is probably accompanied by salivation . . . By measuring saliva flow in response to presentation of stimuli paired with food, Pavlov was probably studying lateral hypothalamic activity almost as directly as if he had a microelectrode there to record action potentials.

If salivation, or salivary response to a palatable food, can be equated, for purposes of speculation, with 'urge to eat', or 'lateral hypothalamic activity', then anything which inhibits salivary response without at the same time having a direct pharmacological action on salivation can be viewed as an anorexigenic agent or satiety agent (assuming proper controls, of course). The most obvious physiological satiety agent is calories, especially in the form of glucose. The study by Wooley, Wooley, and Woods[20] which used amount of salivation elicited by a palatable food as a measure of 'urge to eat' is one of the very few to demonstrate that calories have any effect at all in short-term regulation; what it showed was that the duration of post-meal inhibitory processes are a function of calories. (This is in agreement with Le Magnen[60] who demonstrated, using rats on an *ad lib.* feeding schedule, that the size of a meal is positively correlated with the length of the post-meal interval, but is not related to the length of time since the last meal. So, calories determine when the next meal will be initiated.) An earlier study[66] validated, under several different conditions, the use of this measure with humans.

Thus, salivary response to a palatable food stimulus appears to be a good measure of physiological hunger as a function of deprivation. Because it appears a good measure of the urge to eat, experiments can be designed to determine whether or not a procedure designed to temper appetite (the urge to eat) is effective. For example, Stuart[67] instructed obese patients to eat more slowly. He writes:

> This step . . . helps the patient to derive more enjoyment from his food so that he can replace quantity with quality in his eating. Rapid eating not only leads to indigestion, but it also obviates the possibility for full enjoyment of the taste and aroma of food. By eating more slowly, the patient can improve his digestion and learn to savor his food. He may eventually achieve a *normal state* of satiation with less food intake (our italics).

Stuart's technique was validated (in the study, described earlier) by Wooley, Wooley, and Turner[31] who found that salivary responses elicited by a dessert food stimulus were greater after meals eaten quickly than ones eaten slowly. This effect could have been caused by the greater amount or oral stimulation involved in eating a meal slowly than in eating it rapidly or by post-ingestional factors (e.g. the rate at which food enters the stomach); both are possible explanations since direct neural connections exist between the hypothalamus, and both oral[68,69] and gastric distension[70,71] receptors.

We are a long way from understanding obesity, in large part because so little is known about the processes of regulation of intake even in normal humans. Analogies drawn from animal research on food regulation and learning theory may provide a useful point of departure.

References

1. Bruch, H. (1973). *Eating Disorders: Obesity, Anorexia Nervosa, and the Person Within.* (New York: Basic Books)

2. Schachter, S. (1967). Cognitive effects on bodily functioning: Studies of obesity and eating. In *Biology and Behavior: Neurophysiology and Emotion,* p. 117 (D. G. Glass, editor) (New York: the Rockefeller University Press and Russel Sage Foundation)
3. Schachter, S. (1968). Obesity and eating. *Science,* **161,** 751
4. Schachter, S. (1971). *Emotion, Obesity and Crime.* (New York: Academic Press)
5. Schachter, S., Goldman, R. and Gordon, A. (1968). Effects of fear, food deprivation, and obesity on eating. *J. Personality Soc. Psychol.,* **10,** 91
6. Singh, D. (1973). Role of response habits and cognitive factors in determination of behavior of obese humans. *J. Personality Soc. Psychol.,* **27,** 220
7. Price, J. M. and Grinker, J. (1973). Effects of degree of obesity, food deprivation, and palatability on eating behavior of humans. *J. Comp. Physiol. Psychol.,* **85,** 265
8. Cabanac, M. and Duclaux, R. (1970). Obesity: Absence of satiety aversity to sucrose. *Science,* **168,** 496
9. Cabanac, M. (1971). Physiological role of pleasure. *Science,* **173,** 1103
10. Wooley, O. W., Wooley, S. C. and Dunham, R. B. (1972). Calories and sweet taste: Effects on sucrose preference in the obese and non-obese. *Physiology and Behavior,* **9,** 765
11. Meyer, J. E. and Pudel, V. (1972). Experimental studies on food-intake in obese and normal weight subjects. *J. Psychosom. Res.,* **16,** 305
12. Spiegel, T. A. (1973). Caloric regulation of food intake in man. *J. Comp. Physiol. Psychol.,* **84,** 24
13. Jordan, H. A. (1969). Voluntary intragastric feeding: Oral and gastric contributions to food intake and hunger in man. *J. Comp. Physiol. Psychol.,* **68,** 498
14. Jordan, H. A. (1973). Physiological control of food intake in man. Paper presented at the Fogarty International Conference on Obesity, Washington, D.C., Oct. 1-3. (In press)
15. Wooley, S. C. (1972). Physiologic versus cognitive factors in short-term food regulation in the obese and non obese. *Psychosom. Med.,* **34,** 62
16. Wooley, O. W., Wooley, S. C. and Dunham, R. B. (1972). Can calories be perceived and do they affect hunger in obese and non obese humans? *J. Comp. Physiol. Psychol.,* **80,** 250

17. Wooley, O. W., Wooley, S. C. and Dunham, R. B. (1974). Calories and hunger: Lack of relationship in absence of sensory cues. (In preparation)
18. Bloom, P. B., Filion, R. D. L., Stunkard, A. J., Fox, S. and Stellar, E. (1970). Gastric and duodenal motility, food intake and hunger measured in man during a twenty-four hour period. *Amer. J. Dig. Dis.,* **18,** 719
19. Stunkard, A. J. and Fox, S. (1971). The relationship of gastric motility and hunger: a summary of the evidence. *Psychosom. Med.,* **33,** 123
20. Wooley, O. W., Wooley, S. C. and Woods, W. A. (1975). Effect of calories on appetite for palatable food in obese and non-obese humans. *J. Comp. Physiol. Psychol.* (In press)
21. Nisbett, R. E. (1968). Taste, deprivation and weight determinants of eating behavior. *J. Personality Soc. Psychol.,* **10,** 107
22. Decke, E. (1971). Effects of taste on the eating behavior of obese and normal persons. Cited in S. Schachter *Emotion, obesity and crime.* (New York: Academic Press)
23. Jackson, D. (1973). Interference proneness and sensitivity to meal palatability in the obese and non-obese. (Unpublished M.A. Thesis, University of Cincinati)
24. Wooley, O. W. (1971). Long-term food regulation in the obese and non-obese. *Psychosom. Med.,* **33,** 436
25. Campbell, R., Hashim, S. A. and Van Itallie, T. B. (1972). Studies of food-intake regulation in man: Responses to variations in nutritive density in lean and obese subjects. *New Engl. J. Med.,* **285,** 1402
26. Bauer, E. (1971). Inhibition of eating in the obese: cognition or guilt? (Comment) *Amer. Psychol.,* **26,** 738
27. Hashim, S. A. and VAn Itallie, T. B. (1965). Studies in norma and obese subjects using a monitored food-dispensing device, *Ann. N. Y. Acad. Sci.,* **131,** 654
28. Wooley, S. C., Tennenbaum, O. and Wooley, O. W. (1974). A naturalistic observation of the influence of palatability on food choices of obese and non-obese. (In preparation)
29. Goldman, R., Jaffa, M. and Schachter, S. (1968). Yom Kippur, Air France, dormitory food, and the eating behavior of obese and normal persons. *J. Personality Soc. Psychol.,* **10,** 117
30. Nisbett, R. E. (1968). Determinants of food intake in obesity. *Science,* **159,** 1254
31. Wooley, O. W., Wooley, S. C., and Turner, K. (1975). The effect of rate of consumption on appetite in the obese and nonobese.

Presented at, and to be published in the proceedings of, *The First International Congress on Obesity,* London, October, 1974.

32. Ross, L. D. (1969). Cue- and cognition-controlled eating among obese and normal subjects. (Unpublished doctoral dissertation, Columbia University)
33. Levitz, L. S. (1973). The susceptibility of human feeding behaviour to external controls. Paper presented at the Fogarty International Conference on Obesity. Washington, D.C., October 1-3 (In press)
34. Johnson, W. G. (1970). The effect of prior taste and food visibility on the food-directed instrumental performance of obese individuals. (Unpublished doctoral dissertation, Catholic University of America)
35. Goldman, R. L. (1968). The effects of the manipulation of the visibility of food on the eating behavior of obese and normal subjects. (Unpublished doctoral dissertation, Columbia University)
36. Shaw, J. C. (1973). The influence of food type and method of presentation on human ingestive behavior. (Unpublished doctoral dissertation, University of Pennsylvania)
37. Stunkard, A. H. and Levitz, L. S. (1973). The influence of caloric density and availability on the food selections of normal and obese subjects. (In preparation)
38. Schachter, S. and Gross, L. P. (1968). Manipulated time and eating behavior. *J. Personality Soc. Psychol.,* **10,** 98
39. Nisbett, R. E. and Storms, M. D. (1974). Cognitive and social determinants of food intake. In *Thought and Feeling: Cognitive Alteration of Feeling States.* (H. S. London R. E. Nisbett, editors) (Chicago: Aldine)
40. Schachter, S. (1971). Some extraordinary facts about obese humans and rats. *Amer. Psychol.,* **26,** 129
41. Rodin, J. (1973). Effects of distraction on performance of obese and normal subjects. *J. Comp. Physiol. Psychol.,* **83,** 68
42. Pliner, P. L. (1973). Effects of cue salience on the behavior of obese and normal subjects. *J. Abnorm. Psychol.,* **82,** 226
43. Pliner, P. L. (1973). Effect of external cues on the thinking behavior of obese and normal subjects. *J. Abnorm. Psychol.,* **82,** 233
44. Singh, D., Swanson, J., Letz, R. and Sanders, K. (1973). Performance of obese humans on transfer of training and reaction time tests. *Psychosom. Med.,* **35,** 240
45. Cabanac, M., Duclaux, R. and Spector, N. H. (1971). Sensory

feedback in regulation of body weight: Is there a ponderostat? *Nature,* **229,** 125

46. Grinker, J. and Hirsch, J. (1972). Metabolic and behavioral correlates of obesity. In CIBA Foundation Symposium 8 (new series), Physiology, emotion and psychosomatic illness. p. 349 (Amsterdam: Associated Scientific)
47. Glucksman, M. L. and Hirsch, J. (1968). The response of obese patients to weight reduction: A clinical evaluation of behavior. *Psychosom. Med.,* **30,** 1
48. Glucksman, M. L. and Hirsch, J. (1969). The response of obese patients to weight reduction: III. The perception of body size. *Psychosom. Med.,* **31,** 1
49. Glucksman, M. L., Hirsch, J., McCully, R. S., Barron, B. A. and Knittle, J. L. (1968). The response of obese patients to weight reduction: II. A quantitative evaluation of behavior. *Psychosom. Med.,* **30**, 359
50. Grinker, J., Hirsch, J. and Levin, B. (1973). The affective responses of obese patients to weight reduction: A differentiation based on age at onset of obesity. *Psychosom. Med.,* **35,** 57
51. Nisbett, R. E. (1972). Hunger, obesity, and the ventromedial hypothalamus. *Psychol. Rev.,* **79,** 433
52. Hervey, G. R. (1969). Regulation of energy balance. *Nature,* **222,** 629
53. Jordan, H. A. (1973). In defence of body weight. *Amer. Diet Ass.,* **62,** 17
54. Sclafani, A. and Kluge, L. (1974). Food motivation and body weight levels in hypothalamic hyperphagic rats: A dual lipostat model of hunger and appetite. *J. Comp. Physiol. Psychol.,* **86,** 28
55. Valenstein, E. S. (1966). The anatomical locus of reinforcement. *In Progress in Physiological Psychology,* I. (E. Stellar and J. M. Sprague, editors) (New York: Academic Press)
56. Rozin, P. and Kalat, J. W. (1971). Specific hungers and poison avoidance as adaptive specializations of learning. *Psychol. Bull.,* **78,** 459
57. Revusky, S. H. and Garcia, J. (1970). Learned associations over long delays. *The Psychology of Learning and Motivation: Advances in Research and Theory,* IV (C. H. Bower and J. T. Spence, editors) (New York: Academic Press)
58. Le Magnen, Jacques. (1967). Habits and food intake. *Handbook of Physiology.* Vol. 1, Section 6. (C. F. Code and W. Heidel, editors) (Washington, D. C.: American Physiological Society)

59. Lepkovsky, S. (1973). Newer concepts in the regulation of food intake. *Amer. J. Clin. Nutr.*, **26,** 271
60. Le Magnen, J. (1969). Peripheral and systemic actions of food in the caloric regulation of intake. *Ann. N. Y. Acad. Sci.,* **157,** 1126
61. Jacobs, H. L. and Sharma, K. N. (1969). Taste versus calories: Sensory and metabolic signals in the control of food intake. *Ann. N. Y. Acad. Sci.,* **157,** 1084
62. Silverstone, J. T. (1967). The measurement of hunger in relation to food intake. Proceedings VIIth Internat. Cong. Nutrition Hamburg, **2,** 51
63. Stunkard, A. and Koch, C. (1964). The interpretation of gastric motility. I. Apparent bias in the reports of hunger by obese persons. *Arch. Gen. Psychiat.,* **11,** 74
64. Stunkard, A. (1959). Obesity and the denial of hunger. *Psychosom. Med.,* **4,** 281
65. Teitelbaum, P. (1971). The encephalization of hunger. In *Progress in Physiological Psychology,* IV (E. Stellar and J. M. Sprague, editors) (New York: Academic Press)
66. Wooley, S. C. and Wooley, O. W. (1973). Salivation to the sight and thought of food: A new measure of appetite. *Psychosom. Med.,* **35,** 136
67. Stuart, R. B. (1967). Behavioral control of overeating. *Behav. Res. Ther.,* **5,** 357
68. Sharon, I. M. (1965). Sensory properties of food and their function during feeding. *Food Technology,* **19,** 35
69. Kare, M. R. (1969). Digestive functions of taste stimuli. *Olfaction and Taste: Proceedings of the Third International Symposium,* p. 586 (C. Pfaffmann, editor) (New York: The Rockefeller University Press)
70. Anand, B. K. and Pillai, R. V. (1967). Acitivity of single neurons in the hypothalamic feeding centres: Effect of gastric distension. *J. Physiol.* (*London*), **192,** 63
71. Paintal, A. S. (1954). A study of gastric stretch receptors: Their role in the peripheral mechanisms of satiation of hunger and thirst. *J. Physiol.* (*London*), **126,** 255

5

Dietary Treatment of Obesity

A. N. Howard

Success of any diet therapy depends on many factors other than the diet itself, which is often a minor consideration. Without strong motivation, interest of the physician or his assistant, frequent attendance at clinics, the outlook for the patient can be very poor. Nevertheless, one can speculate on the maximum amount of weight loss which can be achieved[1]. Assuming that the loss of lean body mass is small, and that an average patient requires 2500 kcal/day, the weekly calorie deficit on total starvation would be 17 500 kcalories. Each kg of fat is equivalent to approximately 9000 kcalories so that the maximum weight loss could not be greater than 2 kg (4.4 lb) per week. On a diet of 1250 kcal/day, the theoretical loss is half this, namely 1 kg/week. Similar calculations can be made for diets of other calorific values. Since most diets are low in carbohydrate, the initial one to two weeks is accompanied by a loss of body water of about 3 kg; a factor of some psychological importance for the patient[4] (see Chapter 1).

It is general experience that many subjects, even when under control conditions in a metabolic ward, do not achieve this maximum rate of loss. After a time the rate becomes progressively slower. One of the reasons for this is that during caloric restriction energy expenditure decreases by 15-30% (Figure 5.1)[2-4]. The body becomes more efficient in converting available calories from fat into energy. Under normal conditions much of the high energy intermediate ATP is obtained by the glycerophosphate cycle in the cytoplasm, which is a wasteful process compared with mitochondrial oxidation. Caloric restriction leads to

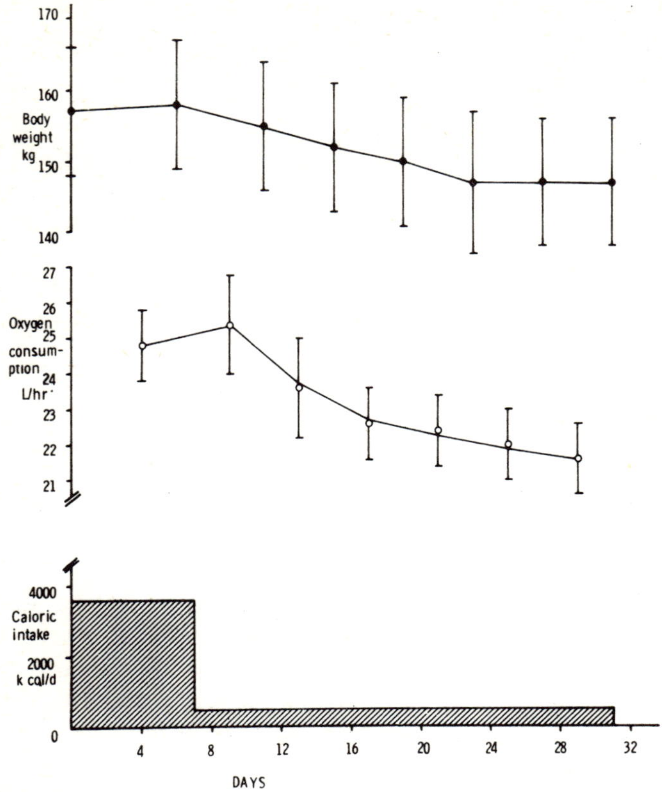

FIGURE 5.1 Effect of calorie intake on body weight and energy expenditure in six obese patients[3]

decreased activity of the enzymes of the glycerophosphate cycle and the alternative more efficient mitochondrial pathway is used and less body heat is generated. Presumably, this is an adaptive mechanism whereby the organism conserves its available energy. Thus, the value of food calories may vary according to food intake and that predictive weight losses may be overestimated.

The results of treatment are often dismal. Glennon (1966) reports that in about 200 subjects who were 50% above their ideal weight, only one patient reached his ideal weight, twelve lost 40 lb and twenty-four 20 lb in a twelve-month follow-up period. Other workers report equally poor results[5,6]. An obvious contributory factor is the loss of motivation by the patient who usually anticipates a greater weight loss than can be achieved and who becomes disappointed with his progress with time. An important factor is therefore the early education of the patient in this respect. Since the fastest weight loss is seen with starvation therapy, and this has received much attention during recent years, it is intended to review this subject first.

STARVATION THERAPY

Modern work stems from the enthusiastic report of Bloom[7] on the use of starvation therapy, which stimulated many other workers to examine this type of treatment[8-11] and the subject has been extensively reviewed[12-16]. The idea is not new and dates back to at least 1915[17]. Opinions differ regarding the effectiveness of this therapy[10,18]. Its protagonists argue that it is successful in reducing the weight of severely affected patients for whom all other pharmacological and dietary measures have failed[19,20]. Since, without exception, these people are greatly at risk, such extreme measures are warranted. Its antagonists point out the danger of depriving the human body of protein, carbohydrates and minerals for excessively long periods of several months[10]. It can carry high risk of fatalities; several deaths have been reported from cardiovascular events[21-25]. One twenty-year-old girl, who died after undergoing starvation for thirty weeks, showed at autopsy histological loss and fragmentation of the myofibrils of the myocardium[24]. Other deaths have been associated with glomerulo-nephritis, lactic acidosis[26] and acute volvulus[27]. As Hartmann and Schmidt concluded in 1967[28], 'until the metabolic effects of prolonged fasting have been thoroughly investigated, the routine use of this method is not recommended'.

During starvation man undergoes a series of metabolic adaptions in order to derive energy from adipose tissue and to conserve as efficiently as possible his protein reserves[29,30]. Glucose is excluded from most tissues and free fatty acids are used as fuel instead. Lipid-derived calories are shuttled to peripheral glycolytic tissues which, in turn, sends lactate back to the liver for resynthesis to glucose. Another, and possibly the most important adaptation, is that of brain to utilise the keto acids, thereby sparing glucose and in turn, body protein. During the first few days of fasting, the blood levels of glucose and insulin are diminished, whereas free fatty acid levels are increased. These levels then remain stable for several weeks if fasting continues.

Weight loss and body composition

The first week of treatment leads to a massive drop in weight of 5-6 kg (Figure 5.2)[8]. This is caused primarily by a loss of intestinal contents and body water[31,32]. Thereafter, a gradual decline of about 2-3 kg/week is seen with a tendency for the rate to decrease with time. Much of this loss is due to lean body mass rather than fat. In fact, the ratio of lean body mass to fat which is lost has been estimated as 6.5: 3.5[33] the magnitude of which was confirmed by others[34-39]. Starvation has been criticised on the grounds that loss in fat is no greater than can be achieved on a 800 kg conventional hospital diet[40]. In a key experiment, Ball *et al.* (1967) alternated a conventional 800 kcal hospital diet with complete

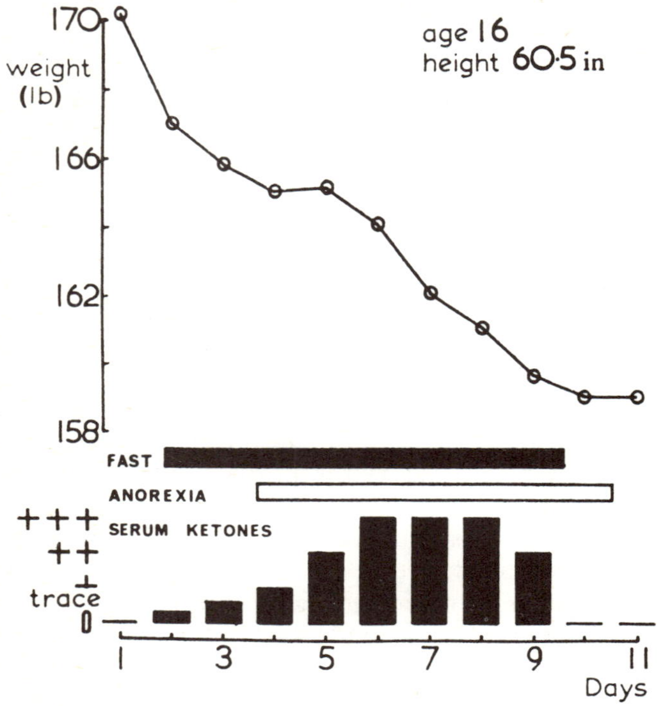

FIGURE 5.2 Starvation therapy in obesity[8]

starvation[36]. As shown in Figure 5.3, the loss in fat tissue was no greater in starvation but there was a considerable loss of lean body mass. However, the excessive nitrogen excretion in the early stages diminishes progressively, such that by thirty days the loss is equivalent to about 25 g/day of protein or 125 g lean body mass (assuming that tissue contains 80% water).

The pathological consequences of this continual loss of nitrogen are not difficult to predict and have all been observed. Serum protein[41] and fibrinogen fall[42]; anaemia develops, caused by a reduction of haemoglobin to 8 g/100 ml and red cells to 3 million/mm [3,43]. Concomitant with this is a significant neutropaenia. Although these latter effects could be due to a deficiency of folic acid or vitamin B12, the

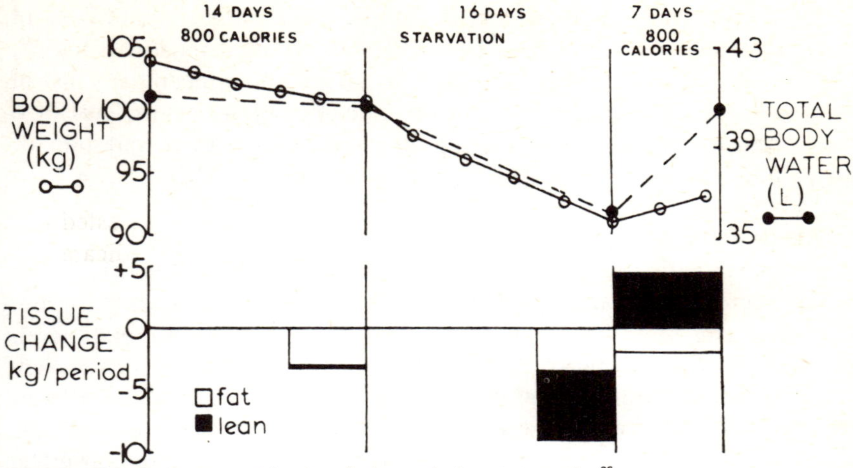

FIGURE 5.3 Body composition in calorie restriction or starvation[36]

abnormalities were not improved by supplements of these vitamins, but only by protein. Liver biopsy samples have revealed focal necrosis, periportal infiltrates and fibrosis[44,45].

Considerable changes occur in amino acid metabolism with plasma alanine becoming greatly decreased[46]. This may be an important component in the regulatory mechanism whereby hepatic gluconeogenesis is diminished and protein catabolism is minimised in prolonged starvation. Hydroxyproline excretion is also increased[47,48]. Since this is an amino acid unique to collagen and sclero-proteins, its metabolism is a reflection of an increased collagen turnover. There is a difference of opinion as to whether bone protein or collagenous supporting structures of fat and other tissues are the chief source of this loss[49,50]. Alopaecia commonly occurs in both men and women.

Electrolytes

Starvation leads to a continuous loss of all electrolytes[51], especially during the initial two weeks. Of these, sodium and potassium are excreted in very high amounts[52-60] and the situation is analogous to hyper-aldosteronism[61]. Such a view is strengthened by the finding of an increased secretion rate and increased urinary excretion of aldosterone[62] (not confirmed by others[63]). Also, the edema which also accompanies starvation contributed to the rise in aldosterone production and possibly of anti-diuretic hormone[64]. A drop in serum sodium occurs after seven weeks and hypokalaemia is evident[65,66]. Diuresis accompanies the loss of sodium and potassium. Postural hypotension is a frequent symptom and may reflect the low levels of serum electrolytes[67].

After forty days of starvation, the loss of magnesium is about 20% of the total body pool[68]. Likewise the urinary excretion of calcium is high[69], particularly during the second to the fifth week and a mean daily loss of about 0.5 g calcium occurs[70]. Serum calcium falls to a low level of 8 mg/100 ml. Neuromuscular symptoms attributable to magnesium or calcium deficiency have not been reported however[71].

Ketosis and acidosis

During starvation all patients develop primary metabolic acidosis, which may occur rapidly and become severe[72] but later disappears[73]. Serum ketones rise after one or two days and eventually reach high levels (Figure 5.2)[8,74]. Urinary ketones are abundant and provide an excellent marker for determining the subject's adherence to the fast[75]. However, there is no evidence that the severe ketosis exerts any deleterious effects. Indeed, according to Bloom (1959) aceto acetic acid has a similar effect to alcohol and may explain the high state of euphoria which most patients exhibit whilst undergoing therapy[7]. It has been suggested that ketosis may be the cause of anorexia[76] but control studies indicate that there is no correlation between the degree of ketosis and absence of hunger when starvation is compared with other conventional diets[77,78].

Uric acid

Serum uric acid rises to high levels (*ca.* 15 mg/100 ml) and may be a cause for some concern[79]. Drenick (1967)[67] states that acute gouty attacks can occur among patients with a past history of gout and, in common with other authors recommends the use of a xanthine oxidase inhibitor such as allopurinol[80,81]. However, this is not the experience of all, since out of forty-two obese patients, Runcie and Thomson[82] found that none developed acute gout, even including one patient with a past history of it.

Hormone function

Since the sole source of energy is adipose tissue, the activity of the adrenal glands are of some importance since adrenal hormones play an important part in lipolysis (see Chapter 2). Free fatty acids are known to rise dramatically[83-85] in acute starvation and stabilise after about fifteen days, and both serum cholesterol[86] and triglycerides fall[87-89]. With acute starvation, catecholamines are increased in adipose tissue[90], cortisol secretion rate declines and 17-hydroxysteroids[91-93] in urine decrease but there is no effect of starvation on adrenocorticol function[94].

Studies on thyroid function reveal no change in protein bound iodine or serum thyroxine. Because of altered liver function, the thyroxine binding power of the serum proteins is diminished leading to increased free thyroxine, insufficient, however, to depress pituitary activity[95].

Plasma growth hormone increases to a peak after ten days and then stabilises to about twice the initial values[96]. Serum insulin falls to about half[97] and excretion diminishes[98] in response to a glucose load but insulin secretion is normal[99]. Glucose tolerance is reduced in the non-diabetic obese[100-105] but not in the diabetic[106]. However, these changes are purely a reflection of the body's adaptation to lack of glucose.

The pituitary gonadal axis remains intact and unaffected[107].

Renal function

Glomerular filtration rate is reduced even with sodium chloride supplements[108]. The average serum creatinine value is elevated and endogenous creatinine clearance lowered[109]. Estimations of urinary proteins suggest impairment of the 'tubular' type but renal function is rapidly restored by refeeding[110]. It is recommended that starvation should be used with caution in patients with impaired renal function.

Intestinal function

Fasting for up to twenty-eight days produced no observable histological changes in the intestinal mucosa[111]. However, transient changes in the metabolism of the jejunal mucosa have been noted including reduced values for certain enzymes and an impaired gastric secretory response to histamine[112]. Although the absorption rates of amino acids[113,114] and calcium[115] are diminished, xylose and oleic acid absorption is unimpaired[116]. Turnover and excretion of bile acids falls to very low levels but returns to normal after refeeding[117].

Success of treatment

Although there is no doubt that weight reduction can readily be achieved by fasting, short periods of treatment offer no advantage over a more conventional diet[8,79,118-124] and should only be employed if there is a pressing indication for temporary weight reduction. Results with longer term starvation are more encouraging, but variable[124-128]. Approximately 50% of patients maintained or bettered their decreased weight loss in three separate studies but at two other centres patients regained weight promptly after cessation of treatment[124,126]. The explanation of the failure rate is simple. It is not difficult to starve in hospital but virtually impossible at home where there is plenty of food available[128]. A greater success rate has been found among patients who are able to achieve a body weight within 20% of the ideal. Presumably, these patients are more strongly motivated than others and have a greater incentive to succeed.

Conclusions

Starvation therapy for weight loss has been used successfully by numerous investigators, chiefly for patients who are refractory to all other methods of treatment. Providing therapy is continued over at least several months a high proportion of successes can be achieved. However, there are many problems and disadvantages. Firstly, it is expensive because the hazards of treatment require the patient to be hospitalised throughout, not only to ensure compliance with treatment, but also to monitor the many biochemical parameters which can show severe abnormalities. These include depletion of essential nutrients, such as protein and minerals, electrolyte imbalance, acidosis and ketosis, hyperuricaemia, postural hypotension, wasting of lean body mass, cardiac irregularities, anaemia and other symptoms, such as increased tendency to gout and alopaecia. All these changes are reversible on returning to a normal diet. Thus, the chief duty of the physician is to monitor such abnormalities to minimise the chance of a fatality. Having succeeded in reducing the weight to within 25% of normal, the chances of maintaining weight loss are evens. As Munro[16] points out 'there remains an urgent need for improved psychological or medical selection in order to minimise the high failure rate'.

VERY LOW CALORIE DIETS

The severe metabolic disturbances induced by complete starvation precludes use of this form of treatment routinely in outpatients. Considerable thought has therefore been given by many workers, to a suitable diet that contains the minimum amount of nutrients consistent with normal health. It is clear that such a diet should contain protein (or a source of amino acids), minerals[129-131] and vitamins, and possibly minimal quantities of carbohydrate. Using conventional foods, Drenick (1967) proposed a 500 kcal diet containing chiefly protein. This is not dissimilar to that widely used by Simeons (1954)[132] and described in Table 5.1. Other workers have employed 200 kcal to 600 kcal diets with considerable success[124,133-136].

To achieve nitrogen balance in starvation therapy 40 - 60 g protein is all that is necessary, for example, egg albumin[137] or casein[138]. The chief metabolic abnormalities with this type of protein diet are ketosis and hyperuricaemia and high electrolyte excretion[139,140]. However, the addition of carbohydrate will produce normality in all these parameters,

TABLE 5.1 *Simeons diet (1954)*[132] *consisting of protein 50%, carbohydrate 20%, fat 30%*

Menu for each meal	
Lean meat	100 g
Leaf vegetables	One helping
Unsweetened rusk	One, small
Apple	One
Salt, fluids	*Ad lib.*

although large quantities of protein will also compensate, presumably by conversion of protein to carbohydrate[141]. The optimum diet is one that contains sufficient protein for nitrogen balance and small quantities of carbohydrate to spare protein.

The quantities required to achieve this were estimated by Baird and Howard (1974)[78]. Following two weeks' starvation, patients were placed on diets containing amino acids or proteins, to which increasing quantities of carbohydrate were added. With a carbohydrate-free diet, the amino acid requirement was about 30 g/day (Figure 5.4). Addition of carbohydrate up to 30—45 g/day had a nitrogen sparing effect and the requirement of nitrogen was reduced to about 15 g/day (Figure 5.5). Increasing the carbohydrate further gave no additional nitrogen sparing effect but produced fluid retention in some patients. It was therefore concluded that the optimal formulation for inpatients is one of 180-360

TABLE 5.2 *Effect of composition of diet on serum uric acid (Baird, Parsons and Howard, 1974)*[78]

	Hospital diet 800 kcal	Chemically defined diet 900 kcal	Starvation	Chemically defined diet carbohydrate g/day			
				0	15	30	80
Case No.	Serum uric acid mg/100 ml						
1	9.4	5.9	13.7	9.1	8.0	3.6	4.7
2	8.2	5.2	14.0	7.9	6.3	6.0	7.0
3	6.5	5.6	7.4	6.1	5.9	4.0	4.0
4	4.6	4.6	8.5	7.4	7.1	6.3	6.2
5	6.7	5.8	10.3	10.0	8.5	6.3	5.0
Mean	7.1	5.4	10.8	8.1	7.2	5.2	5.4

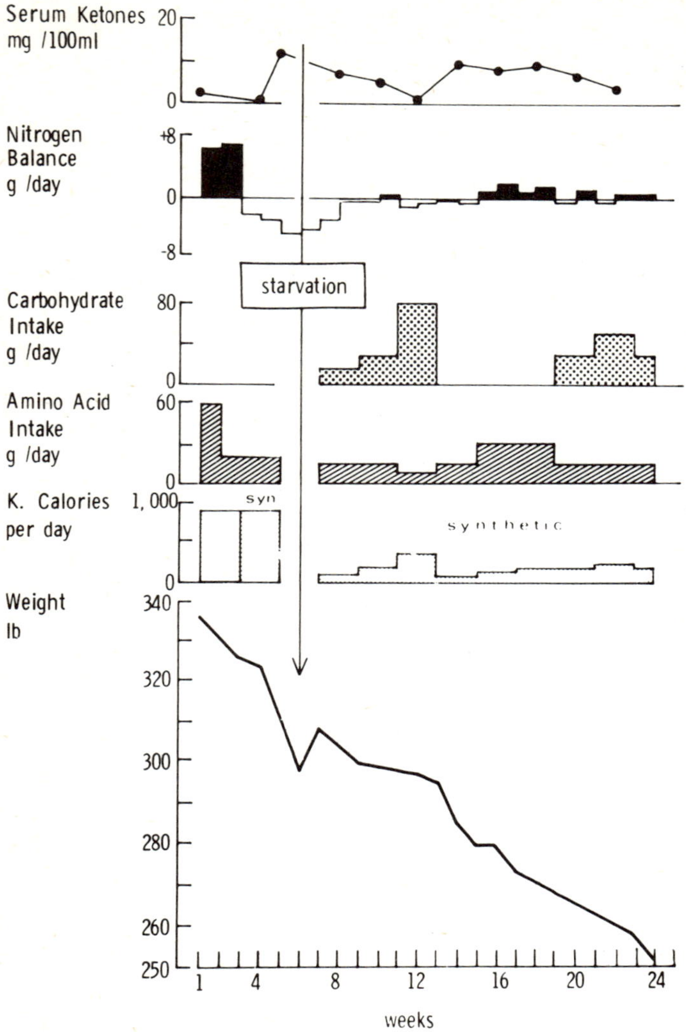

FIGURE 5.4 Effect of very low calorie semi-synthetic diets[78]

kcal that supplies 15 g protein and 30—45 g carbohydrate. Although 80 g/day carbohydrate is needed to abolish ketosis, a moderate degree of serum ketones was well tolerated and with 30 – 45 g of carbohydrate the ketosis is minimal. None of the patients complained of hunger on the formula diets but this was not related to the level of ketones. The hyperuricaemia seen in complete starvation returned to pretreatment levels (Table 5.2). The patients remained in electrolyte balance and no

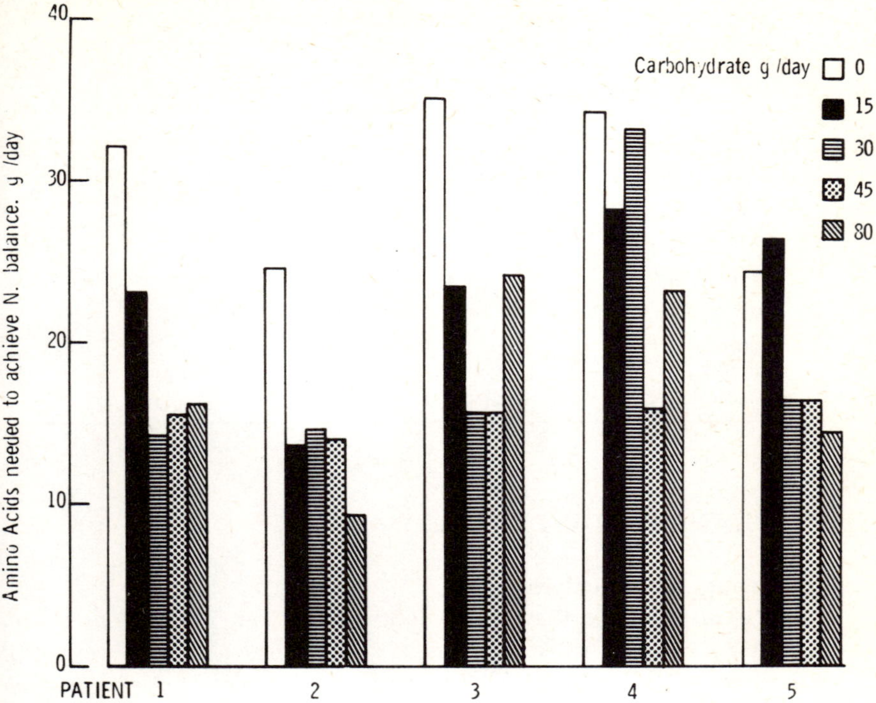

FIGURE 5.5 Effect of carbohydrate intake on amino acids required to achieve nitrogen balance[78]

serious clinical or biochemical abnormalities developed. More recent studies have shown that patients can be trained to consume such a formula diet in hospital and then be released as outpatients, where many continue to lose weight for several months.

The most surprising finding in these studies was the small quantity of protein required which was much less than expected. However, these results are consistent with those of Jourdan *et al.* (1973)[142], who gave a diet containing 25% of the energy required to maintain body weight (about 600 kcal), consisting of carbohydrate but no protein, the equivalent nitrogen loss was about 18 g protein/day.

Conclusions

Very low calorie diets offer a much safer alternative to complete starvation. As shown in Table 5.3, the main disadvantages can be circumvented, whilst the rate of weight loss remains high. Moreover, the procedure need not be expensive since the patient is required to remain in hospital for only a short period. In addition there is little danger of serious biochemical and clinical abnormalities developing.

TABLE 5.3 *Comparison of starvation and very low calorie diets*

Parameter	Starvation	Very low calorie diets (180-360 kcal)
Weight loss	Very good	Very good
Patient acceptance	Poor	Good
Ketosis	Excessive	Minimal
Serum uric acid	High	Normal
Nitrogen balance	Negative	Equilibrium achieved
Water balance	Diuresis	Normal
Electrolyte excretion (K^+, Na^+, Ca^{++})	High negative balance	Equilibrium achieved
Safety	High risk	Theoretically safe

CONVENTIONAL DIET THERAPY

Equivalence of food calories

There is no evidence that over a long period, fat, carbohydrate and protein calories are substantially different. A loss in body weight is dependent on the total caloric deficit. Earlier studies by Kekwick and Pawan (1956) showed that over short periods, weight loss from high carbohydrate diets of 1000 kcal was less than with isocaloric diets of fat and protein. However, these results can be explained purely on changes in body water and not in body fat[143-145]. Patients on high carbohydrate diets can initially be in positive water balance and exhibit sodium retention[146], the mechanism of which is obscure. The situation was clarified by Pilkington *et al.*[147] who gave patients a diet consisting of either 91% fat or 86% carbohydrate (Figure 5.6) alternately. Over periods of at least twenty-four days there was no difference in terms of weight loss between high fat or high carbohydrate diets[148-152].

Confusion has arisen in the past because of the success of the so called 'high fat' diet of Taller (1962)[153] in which obese people were advised to eat as much fat as they wished. However, as Yudkin and Carey (1960)[154] clearly demonstrated, the so called 'high fat' diet is really a low carbohydrate one. Because of carbohydrate restriction, patients allowed a free choice actually consumed less fat than they did normally.

The low carbohydrate-high protein diet

Among dietitians and nutritionists two types of dietary management are common:

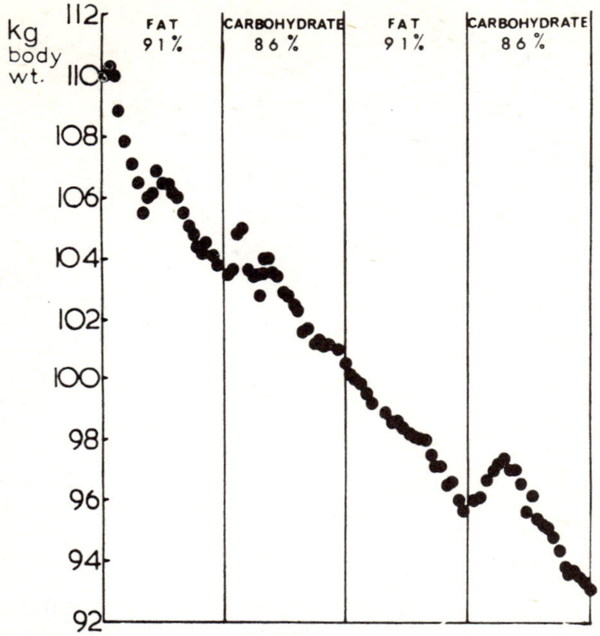

FIGURE 5.6 Effect of composition of diet. Patient given 1000 Kcal fat or carbohydrate[147]

(1) The calorie controlled diet, which the patient is given different menus containing a stated number of calories,
(2) The low carbohydrate diet; in which all foods containing carbohydrate are avoided[155].

In practice, there is often not much difference between the two schemes, since both rely on protein as the chief source of calories. Most diets are in the range of 800—1500 kcal/day[156].

A survey among general practitioners in the United Kingdom revealed that most advised the low carbohydrate diet[157], its great advantage being that it is easy to prescribe and involves no weighing of food by the patient. As shown in Table 5.4, the intake of nutrients of subjects on such a diet of 1750 kcal/day is as good as with a normal diet of 1000 kcal greater[158]. The high protein content ensures that negative nitrogen balance is reduced or completely abolished[36,159-161]. This is important where treatment is likely to be prolonged for several months or even years. A common feature is that the patients' hunger is completely satisfied compared with a diet high in carbohydrate and of the same calorific value[154,162-164]. The reason for the satiety effect is not completely clear but it is known that digestion of protein is much slower

TABLE 5.4 *Nutrient intakes of subjects on a low carbohydrate diet* (Stock and Yudkin, 1970)[158]

	Normal diet	Low carbohydrate diet
Total calories (kcal)	2370	1560
Protein calories	84	83
Fat calories	124	105
Carbohydrate calories	216	67
Vitamin A	2.06 mg	2.07 mg
Carotene	1.0 mg	1.03 mg
Ascorbic acid	70 mg	75 mg
Vitamin D	200 i.u.	310 i.u.
Thiamine	1.13 mg	0.93 mg
Riboflavin	1.66 mg	1.75 mg
Nicotinic acid	13.1 mg	11.0 mg
Calcium	1070 mg	980 mg
Iron	12.8 mg	11.7 mg

than carbohydrate and protein foods often remain in the stomach longer.

Clinical results using a relatively high protein diet are often encouraging in children. Marked improvements can be obtained. As shown in Figure 5.7, a comparison was made between children aged nine to thirteen on a conventional clinic slimming diet moderately high in protein, and in those on a diet very high in protein, using a high protein dietetic loaf[165]. The conventional reducing diet was rather unsuccessful and only small weight losses were achieved. With the very high protein diet, a mean weight loss of 8 lb over several months was achieved and after six months 40% of the children had lost over 12 lb.

Meal frequency

Fabry and his colleagues (1964)[166] analysed a group of 379 Czech men to determine the relationship between frequency of food intake and their percentage overweight (Table 5.5). Those men consuming five or more meals a day were found to have gained less weight than those having three meals a day or less. A study of Czech women by other workers[167] also gave a similar result in the same direction. From these results it was concluded that a greater weight loss might be achieved by slimming diets if taken in several small meals. However, under the conditions of the metabolic ward no difference in effects resulting from changes in meal pattern has been obtained. Bortz and his colleagues (1966)[168].

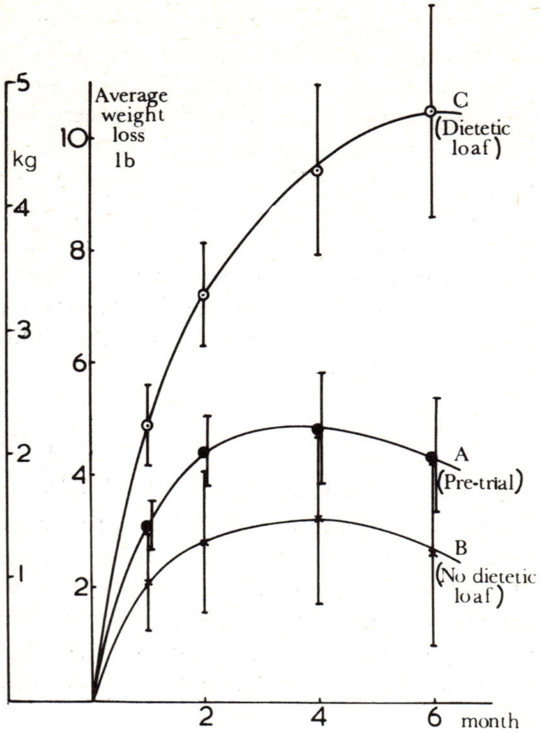

FIGURE 5.7 Weight loss in children receiving a high protein dietetic loaf[165]

using a 600 kcal diet found no difference between one, three and nine feedings a day. Likewise, others obtained similar results with a 1700 kcal diet[169].

In a Scottish study there was no differences in mean weight loss between two and five meals a day of 1000 kcal in outpatients[170-1]. A

TABLE 5.5 *Incidence of overweight and hypocholesterolaemia in Czech men* Fabry *et al.* (1964)[166]

Group	No. meals/day	No. examined	Overweight* (%)	Hyper-cholesterolaemia† (%)
1	2 or less	42	57	51
2	3-4	206	42	35
3	5 or more	38	29	18

**> 10% correct weight

† > 260 mg %

notable finding was that the number of patients adhering to the five meal a day plan was very much less than those on the two meal regime. Nevertheless, a number of patients who had failed to lose weight on the two meals a day regime were successful with five. A similar result was obtained by Debry (1971)[172]. In fifty-two obese subjects, the mean daily weight loss on the same reducing diet, was 78 g for three meals and 142 g for seven meals. However, there was a great individual variation. Out of the twenty-six patients receiving seven meals a day, a greater weight loss was obtained in thirteen and a lesser weight loss in seven. Thus, the 'multi-meal' method may be of value where the conventional three meal a day diet proves ineffective. In some people multi-meals may have a greater appetite suppressing power.

EXERCISE

Energy expenditure of the obese is considerably less than of thin people and the difference can be quite large[173-174]. In a group of high school girls, the average daily expenditure for obese children was 1260 kcal, compared with 1965 kcal for lean subjects[175]. Other studies show that obese people spend less time on their feet and more time in bed[176]. Although obese people claim to eat no more food than thin people, it is not clear to what extent inactivity has led to obesity rather than the reverse.

A number of studies show that exercise is beneficial in increasing weight loss. In one of these[177], five overweight men, aged thirty-five to forty-six years entered a training programme and gradually worked up to being able to cover three miles in thirty minutes thrice weekly. The decrease in weight, due to exercise alone, after sixteen weeks, averaged 4.5 kg. Likewise, obese college women[178], when exercised on a treadmill and bicycle ergometer four days a week for one hour and receiving a 1200 kcal diet, showed increased weight loss over those given the diet alone.

From theoretical considerations, considerable physical activity is needed to make an impression on body fat. For example, it takes three rounds of golf to expend the equivalent of 1 kg adipose tissue. On the other hand, walking an extra one or two miles daily could cause an annual weight loss of nearly 6 kg, providing there was no increased food consumption[16]. Other evidence suggests that exercise can increase metabolic activity, particularly after the ingestion of food[179]. Consuming 1000 kcal for breakfast has a thermic effect and increases oxygen consumption by 10%. The additional effect of exercise is of the same magnitude. The general conclusion is that not only is exercise beneficial but particularly so after eating a large meal, provided that there are no cardiovascular contra-indications.

GROUP THERAPY

With inpatients under strict supervision there is no difficulty in obtaining weight reduction. It is with outpatients that difficulties arise and there are many failures. Among many important factors for success are the skill and personality of the dietitian, but frequent visits are probably of greater importance [180-1]. Education of the patient in new dietary habits can also be achieved by his taking meals at the hospital as an outpatient, followed later by regular weekly consultations with the physician.

In practice such ideas are not likely to be welcomed enthusiastically by the already over-worked physician, and group therapy seems to be a logical compromise. In a recent experiment[182], a comparison was made between eighteen patients attending an outpatients clinic monthly and a similar number with comparable initial weight of people meeting weekly in a comparable group each being given the same dietary instructions. As shown in Figure 5.8 a loss in weight over fourteen weeks in the group was almost double that of the outpatients and almost equivalent to the ideal achieved by patients under strict supervision. During recent years there has been a considerable expansion in the number of commercial slimming clubs, and their popularity is some proof of their success. A recent survey[183] showed that members of slimming clubs stayed an average of twenty-six weeks and lost an average of 9 kg (11% body weight). This is considered more successful than that usually achieved by general practitioners.

CONCLUSIONS

The failure of conventional dietary treatment in a large number of severely obese people is a major problem for the physician. Long-term starvation in hospital is a procedure which is highly effective but not without considerable risk. Because of the expense involved, the treatment cannot become widespread. Newer developments with very low calorie semi-synthetic diets offer a logical alternative whereby the patient can ultimately be treated as an outpatient, with a much greater degree of safety and with almost the same rapid weight loss. Even then, the final outcome may be disappointing since 50% of the grossly obese rapidly increase their weight again after cessation of treatment. This is a problem which so far no one has successfully tackled.

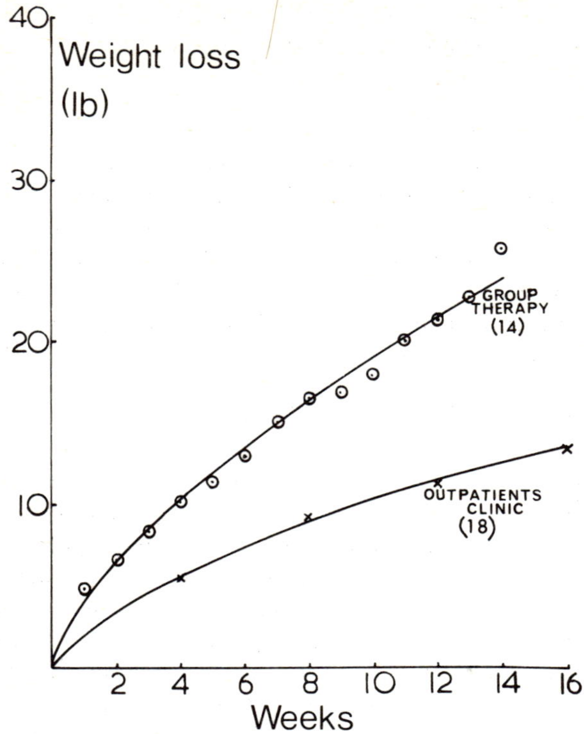

FIGURE 5.8 Group therapy and weight loss using a 1000 Kcal diet[182]

Among conventional methods the low carbohydrate diet proves the most popular among physicians. To ensure success, the patient must be seen regularly and realistic advice given about the anticipated weight loss. Group therapy by one of the commercial 'slimming clubs' has proved a boon to the overworked doctor when other methods fail. Finally the benefit of exercise cannot be over-stressed.

However, the long-term treatment of obesity can best be achieved by a re-education of the patient in his dietary habits. Whatever the treatment and however initially successful, the ultimate goal has to be continuing maintenance of body weight at a desirable level.

REFERENCES

1. Bortz, W. M. (1968). Predictability of weight loss. *J. Amer. Med. Assoc.,* **204,** 101
2. Apfelbaum, M., Bostarron, J. and Brigant, L. (1969). Reduction in basal oxygen consumption under the influence of energy

restriction in subjects in N balance. *Rev. Franc. Etudes Clin. Biol.,* **14,** 361

3. Bray, G. A. (1969). Effect of caloric restriction on energy expenditure in obese patients. *Lancet,* **ii,** 397
4. Bray, G. A. (1970). The myth of diet in the management of obesity. *Amer. J. Clin. Nutrition,* **23,** 1141
5. Stunkard, A. (1959). Results of treatment for obesity. *Arch. Intern. Med.,* **103,** 79
6. Liebermeister, H., Jahnke, K., Voss, H. J., Englhardt, A. and Probst, G. (1968). Initial and late results of diet treatment of obesity. *Deutsch. Med. Wochenschr.,* **93,** 2149
7. Bloom, W. L. (1959). Fasting as an introduction to the treatment of obesity. *Metabolism,* **8,** 214
8. Duncan, G. C., Jenson, W. K., Fraser, R. L. and Cristofori, F. C. (1962). Correction and control of intractable obesity. *J. Amer. Med. Ass.,* **181,** 309
9. Duncan, G. C., Jenson, W. K., Cristofori, F. C. and Schlers, G. L. (1963). Intermittent fasts in the correction and control of intractable obesity. *Amer. J. Med. Sci.,* **245,** 515
10. Drenick, E. J., Swendseid, M. E., Tuttle, S. G. and Blahd, W. H. (1964). Prolonged starvation as treatment for severe obesity. *J. Amer. Med. Ass.,* **187,** 100
11. Van Riet, H. G., Schwarz, F. and Der Kinderen, P. J. (1964). Metabolic observations during the treatment of obese patients by periods of total starvation. *Metabolism,* **13,** 291
12. Swanson, D. W. and Dinello, F. (1969). Therapeutic starvation in obesity. *Dis. Nervous System,* **30,** 669
13. Gibinski, K. (1969). Starvation treatment of obesity. *Polski Tyg. Lek.,* **24,** 951
14. Wildenhoff, K. E. and Sørensen, N. S. (1969). Absolute fasting in the treatment of obesity. Recent aspects. *Nord. Med.,* **82,** 1197
15. Weinsier, R. L. (1971). Fasting—a review with emphasis on the electrolytes. *Amer. J. Med.,* **50,** 223
16. Munro, J. F. (1973). The management of obesity. *Brit. J. Hosp. Med.,* **10** (1), 8
17. Folin, O. and Dennis, W. (1915). On starvation and obesity, with special reference to acidosis. *J. Biol. Chem.,* **21,** 183
18. Conzolazio, C. F., Matoish, L. O., Johnson, H. L., Kryzywicki, H. J., Issac, G. J. and Witt, N. F. (1968). Metabolic aspects of calorie restriction: Hypohydration effects on body weight and blood parameters. *Amer. J. Clin. Nutr.,* **21,** 793

19. Ditschuneit, H., Faulhaber, J. D., Beil, I. and Pfeiffer, E. F. (1970). Metabolic changes on complete fasting. *Internist,* **11,** 176
20. Ditschuneit, H. (1971). Metabolism in obesity and in complete fasting. *Medizin und Ernährung,* **12,** 169
21. Spencer, I.O.B. (1968). Death during therapeutic starvation for obesity. *Lancet,* **i,** 1288
22. Hermann, L. S. and Iversen, M. (1968). Death during therapeutic starvation. *Lancet,* **ii,** 217
23. Kahan, A. (1968). Death during therapeutic starvation. *Lancet,* **i,** 1378
24. Garnett, E. S., Barnard, D. L., Ford, J., Goodbody, R. A. and Woodehouse, M. A. (1969). Gross fragmentation of cardiac myofibrils after therapeutic starvation for obesity. *Lancet,* **i,** 914
25. Lawlor, T. (1968). Death during therapeutic starvation. *Lancet,* **ii,** 44
26. Cubberley, P. J., Polster, S. A. and Schulman, C. L. (1965). Lactic acidosis and death after the treatment of obesity by fasting. *New Engl. J. Med.,* **272,** 1965
27. Runcie, J. and Thomson, T. J. (1970). Prolonged starvation — a dangerous procedure? *Brit. Med. J.,* **3,** 432
28. Hartmann, G. and Schmid, R. (1967). Prolonged fasting as a form of treatment of obesity. *Deutsch. Med. Wochenschr.,* **92,** 1663
29. Cahill, G. F. (Jr.) (1970). Starvation in man. *New Engl. J. Med.,* **282,** 668
30. Flatt, J. P. and Blackburn, G. L. (1974). The metabolic fuel regulatory system implications for protein-sparing therapies during caloric deprivation and disease. *Amer. J. Clin. Nutr.,* **27,** 175
31. Azar, G. J. and Bloom, W. L. (1963). Similarities of carbohydrate deficiency and fasting. *Arch. Intern. Med.,* **112,** 338
32. Bloom, W. L. and Azar, G. J. (1963). Similarities of carbohydrate deficiency and fasting. *Arch Intern. Med.,* **112,** 333
33. Benoir, F. L., Martin, R. L. and Watten, R. H. (1965). Changes in body composition during weight reduction in obesity. *Ann. Intern. Med.,* **63,** 604
34. Apfelbaum, M. (1966). Changes in major physiological com-

partments during fasting. *Cahiers Nutrition Dietetique,* **1,** No. 4, 35

35. Apfelbaum, M., Bost-Sarron, J., Brigant, L. and Dupin, H. (1967). Composition of the weight lost on a water diet. Effects of protein supplementation. *Gastroenterologia,* **108,** 121
36. Ball, M. F., Canary, J. J. and Kyle, L. H. (1967). Comparative effects of caloric restriction and total starvation on body composition in obesity. *Ann. Int. Med.,* **67,** 60
37. Gilder, H., Cornell, G. N., Grafe, W. R., Macfarlane, J. R., Asaph, J. W., Stubenbord, W. T., Watkins, G. M., Rees, J. R. and Thorbjarnarson, B. (1967). Components of weight loss in obese patients subjected to prolonged starvation. *J. Appl. Physiol.,* **23,** 304
38. Seager, B. C. (1969). Body composition in early starvation as measured by a pneumatic body volumeter and whole-body potassium 40. *Dissertation Absts. Internat.* (*B*), **30,** 365B
39. Ball, M. F., Canary, J. J. and Kyle, L. H. (1970). Tissue changes during intermittent starvation and caloric restriction as treatment for severe obesity. *Arch. Intern. Med.,* **125**, 62
40. Blondheim, S., Kaufmann, N. A. and Stein, M. (1965). Comparison of fasting and 800-1000 calorie diet in treatment of obesity. *Lancet,* **i,** 250
41. Skugarevskii, A. F., Vier, V. G., Skugarevskaya, E. I., Donskoi, D. I. and Korzhevskaya, I. L. (1971). Changes in some metabolic values during therapeutic fasting. In *Biokhimiya i Patokhimiya Obmena Veshchestv i Mekhanizmy Ego Regulyatsii,* p. 124 (Minsk: "Belarus")
42. Fekete, T., Dutu, A., Podut, E. and Deleanu, M. (1971). Changes in coagulation and fibrinolysis during treatment of obesity by starvation. *Clujul Medical,* **44,** 131
43. Drenick, E. J. and Alvarez, L. C. (1971). Neutropenia in prolonged fasting. *Amer. J. Clin. Nutr.,* **24,**859
44. Rozental, P., Biava, C., Spencer, H. and Zimmerman, H. J. (1967). Liver morphology and function tests in obesity and during total starvation. *Amer. J. Digest. Dis.,* **12,** 198
45. Drenick, E. J., Simmons, F. and Murphy, J. F. (1970). Effect on hepatic morphology of treatment of obesity by fasting, reducing diets and small bowel bypass. *New Engl. J. Med.,* **282,** 829
46. Felig, P., Owen, O. E., Wahren, J. and Cahill, G. F. (1969). Amino acid metabolism during prolonged starvation. *J. Clin. Invest.,* **48,** 584

47. Bell, N. H. (1969). Observations concerning the effects of fasting on collagen metabolism in man. *J. Clin. Endocrinol.*, **29**, 338
48. Ball, M. F., Canary, J. J. and Houck, J. C. (1972). Studies of the hydroxyprolinuria of fasting. *J. Clin. Endocrinol. Metab.*, **35**, 416
49. Brown, H., Milner, A., Kennedy, J. and Delena, S. (1968). Hydroxyproline excretion during starvation of obese subjects. *Metabolism*, **17**, 345
50. Litvak, J., Wortsman, J., Pumarino, H. and Armendaris, R. (1968). Effect of fasting on urinary calcium and hydroxyproline excretion in obesity. *J. Clin. Endocrinol.*, **28**, 311
51. Bloom, W. L. and Mitchell, W. (1960). Salt excretion of fasting patients. *Arch. Intern. Med.*, **106**, 321
52. Smith, R. and Drenick, E. J. (1966). Changes in body water and sodium during prolonged starvation for extreme obesity. *Clin. Sci.*, **31**, 437
53. Hamwi, G. J., Mitchell, M. C., Wieland, R. G., Kruger, F. A. and Schachner, S. S. (1967). Sodium and potassium metabolism during starvation. *Amer. J. Clin. Nutrition*, **20**, 897
54. De Divitiis, O., Cerqua, R., Giordano, F., Moro, C. O., Jacono, A. and Mancini, M. (1968). Effects of prolonged fasting on some aspects of water and salt metabolism in obesity in man. *Folia Angiol.*, No. 2, 178
55. Bittnerova, H. and Zvolankova, K. (1968). ^{24}Na distribution space and total exchangeable Na with bodyweight in equilibrium and changes after starvation and after a diet low in energy in obese women. *Ces. Gastroenterol. Vyz.*, **22**, 6
56. Drenick, E. J. (1968). The relation of BSP retention during prolonged fasts to changes in plasma volume. *Metabolism*, **17**, 522
57. Hendrikx, A. and De Moor, P. (1969). Metabolic changes in obese patients during fasting and refeeding. *Acta Clin. Belg.*, **24**, 1
58. Nielsen, S. L., Juhl, E. and Quaade, F. (1969). Metabolic changes during total fasting. *Ugeskr. Loeger*, **131**, 183
59. Kjellberg, J. and Reizenstein, P. (1970). Effect of starvation on body composition in obesity. *Acta Med. Scand.*, **188**, 171
60. Runcie, J. (1971). Urinary sodium and potassium excretion in fasting obese subjects. *Brit. Med. J.*, **2**, 22
61. Hansen, E. L., Hørlyck, E., Grønbaek, P. and Iversen, M. (1967). Hyperaldosteronism following total fasting in obese subjects. *Acta Med. Scand.*, **182**, 65

62. Giocoli, G. (1969). Changes in excretion of aldosterone in urine during absolute starvation in essential obesity. *Ann. 1st. Super. Sanita, Rome,* **5,** 514
63. Smith, R., Ross, E. J. and Marshall-Jones, P. (1969). Aldosterone and sodium excretion in obese subjects on water diet. *Metabolism,* **18,** 700
64. Hermann, L. S., Hansen, N. C., Grønbaek, P. and Iversen, M. (1969). Hyperaldosteronism after weight reduction by complete fasting. *Ugeskr. Loeger,* **131,** 192
65. Mancini, M., Oriente, P., Moro, C. O., Cerqua, R., de Divitiis, O. and Cioffi, L. A. (1968). Blood lipids and total exchangeable Na during prolonged fasting in simple obesity and obesity with diabetes. *Boll. Soc. Ital. Biol. Sper.,* **44,** 2234
66. Lawlor, T. and Wells, D. G. (1969). Metabolic hazards of fasting. *Amer. J. Clin. Nutrition,* **22,** 1142
67. Drenick, E. J. (1967). Weight reduction with low calorie diets. *J. Amer. Med. Ass.,* **202,** 118
68. Drenick, E. J., Hunt, I. F. and Swendseid, M. E. (1969). Magnesium depletion during prolonged fasting of obese males. *J. Clin. Endocrinol.,* **29,** 1341
69. Fromm, G. A., Najenson, H., Degrossi, O., Miseta, O., Pecorini, V. and Farias, E. (1968). Metabolic effects of therapeutic fasting. *Rev. Asoc. Med. Argent.,* **82,** 388
70. Garnett, J., Garnett, E. S., Mardell, R. J. and Barnard, D. L. (1970). Urinary calcium excretion during ketoacidosis of prolonged total starvation. *Metabolism,* **19,** 502
71. Hunt, I. F. (1970). Magnesium studies in obese subjects during fasting and refeeding. *Dissertation Absts. Internat.* (*B*), **30,** 5114B
72. Voigt, K. D., Apostolakis, M. and Jungmann, H. (1967). Studies of metabolism and circulation in total fasting. *Klin. Wochenschr.,* **45,** 924
73. Ross, S. K., Macleod, A., Ireland, J. T. and Thomson, W. S. T. (1969). Acidosis in obese fasting patients. *Brit. Med. J.,* **1,** 380
74. Wildenhoff, K. E., Dalsager, H. H. and Sørensen, N. S. (1969). Ketone bodies in blood and urine of overweight patients treated by absolute fasting. *Nord Med.,* **82,** 1201
75. Gonciarz, Z., Makowski, C. and Krol, Z. (1972). Clinical value of estimating ketones in urine of obese persons treated by starvation. *Polski Tygodnik Lekarski,* **27,** 293
76. Andreoli, C. and Lenzi, G. (1967). Fasting in the treatment of obesity. *Far East Med. J.,* **3,** 20, 22

77. Silverstone, J. E., Stark, J. E. and Buckle, R. M. (1966). Hunger during total starvation. *Lancet,* **i,** 1343
78. Baird, I. McLean, Parsons, R. L. and Howard, A. N. (1974). Clinical and metabolic studies of chemically defined diets in the management of obesity. *Metabolism,* **23,** 645
79. Gilliland, I. C. (1968). Total fasting in the treatment of obesity. *Postgrad. Med. J.,* **44,** 58
80. Munro, J. F., MacCuish, A. C., Goodall, J. A. D., Fraser, J. and Duncan, L. J. P. (1970). Further experience with prolonged thereapeutic starvation in gross refractory obesity. *Brit. Med. J.,* **4,** 712
81. Schatanoff, J., Duncan, T. G. and Duncan, G. G. (1970). Effects of allopurinol on hyperuricemia secondary to fasting. *Metabolism,* **19,** 84
82. Runcie, J. and Thomson, T. J. (1969). Total fasting, hyperuricaemia and gout. *Postgrad. Med. J.,* **45,** 251
83. Bisacchi, U., Morabito, F. and Strazzulla, G. (1966). Mobilisation of unesterified fatty acids during fasting in obese subjects on a reducing diet. *Riv. Clin. Pediat.,* **78,** 494
84. Owen, O. E., Felig, P., Morgan, A. P., Wahren, J. and Cahill, G. F. Jr (1969). Liver and kidney metabolism during prolonged starvation. *J. Clin. Invest.,* **48,** 574
85. Owen, O. E. and Reichard, G. A., Jr. (1971). Human forearm metabolism during progressive starvation. *J. Clin. Invest.,* **50** 1536
86. Spahn, U., Plenert, W. and Pathenheiner, F. (1967). Treatment by fasting in juvenile obesity. 1. Changes of bodyweight during reduced energy intake and absolute fasting. 2. Free fatty acids in serum during drastic restriction of energy and during total starvation. *Ztschr. Kinderheilk,* **100,** 160 **101,** 20
87. Spahn, U. and Plenert, W. (1968). Treatment of obesity in childhood by starvation. 3. Behaviour of serum lipids during drastic restriction of energy and during absolute starvation. *Ztschr. Kingerheilk,* **103,** 13
88. Jackson, I. M. D. (1969). Effect of prolonged starvation on blood lipid levels of obese subjects. *Metabolism,* **18,** 13
89. Voigt, K. D. and Apostolakis, M. (1969). Effect of complete fasting for 20 days on the substrates of carbohydrate and fat metabolism and on enzyme activities in blood. *Klin. Wochenschr.,* **47,** 157
90. Sdrobici, D., Bonaparte, H., Pieptea, R. and Sapatino, V. (1967). The role of the catecholamines in fat mobilisation from

the adipose tissue in fasting obese patients. *Nutritio et Dieta,* **9,** 271

91. Haag, B. L., Reidenberg, M. M., Shuman, C. R. and Channick, B. J. (1967). Aldosterone, 17-hydroxycorticosteroid, 17-ketosteroid, and fluid and electrolyte responses to starvation and selective refeeding. *Amer. J. Med. Sci.,* **254,** 652
92. Azerad, E. (1968). Treatment of obesity by total fasting. *Sem. Hop. Sem. Therap.,* **44,** Th. 338-Th. 341
93. Garces, L. Y., Kenny, F. M., Drash, A. and Taylor, F. H. (1969). Cortisol secretion rate during fasting of obese adolescent subjects. *J. Clin. Endocrinol.,* **28,** 1843
94. Sabeh, G., Alley, R. A., Robbins, T. J., Narduzzi, J. V., Kenny, F. M. and Danowski, T. S. (1969). Adrenocortical indices during fasting in obesity. *J. Clin. Endocrinol.,* **29,** 373
95. Schatz, D. L., Sheppard, R. H., Palter, H. C. and Jaffri, M. H. (1967). Thyroid function studies in fasting obese subjects. *Metabolism,* **16,** 1075
96. Iacono, G., Giudice, N. Del., Chionni, A., Colucci, M., and Palomba, D. (1971). Behaviour of HGH in obese adolescents after prolonged fasting and low-energy diet. *Folia Endocrinologica,* **24,** 235
97. Giudice, N. Del., Ghionni, A., Colucci, M., Palomba, D. and Jacono, G. (1971). Behaviour of HGH in primary obesity and variations after fasting. *Folia Endocrinologica,* **24,** 281
98. Hellier, M. D. (1970). The effects of prolonged starvation and refeeding on 24-hr. urinary insulin levels in obese subjects. *J. Endocrinol.,* **47,** 73
99. Metz, R., Nice, M., Berger, S. and Mako, M. (1968). Preservation of insulin and liver glycogen stores during very long fasts. *J. Lab. Clin. Med.,* **71,** 573
100. Corredor, D. G., Sabeh, G., Mendelsohn, L. V., Wasserman, R. E., Sunder, J. H. and Danowski, T. S. (1969). Enhanced post-glucose hypophosphatemia during starvation therapy of obesity. *Metabolism,* **18,** 754
101. Jackson, I. M. D., McKiddie, M. T. and Buchanan, K. D. (1969). Effect of fasting on glucose and insulin metabolism of obese patients. *Lancet,* **i,** 285
102. Kolanowski, J., Pizarro, M. A., De Gasparo, M., Desmecht, P., Harvengt, C. and Crabbe, J. (1970). Influence of fasting on adrenocortical and pancreatic islet response to glucose loads in the obese. *European J. Clin. Invest.,* **1,** 25
103. Iacono, G., Giudice, N. Del., Ghionni, A., Colucci, M. and

Palomba, D. (1971). Effects of prolonged starvation and of low-energy diet on plasma levels of growth hormone and insulin in obese persons. *Acta Diabetologica Latina,* **8,** 500

104. Jackson, I. M. D., McKiddie, M. T. and Buchanan, K. D. (1971). Influence of blood-lipid levels and effect of prolonged fasting on carbohydrate metabolism in obesity. *Lancet,* **ii,** 450

105. Cravetto, C. A., Favero, A. and Cravario, A. (1973). Metabolic aspects of prolonged fasting in obese subjects. *Folia Endocrinologica,* **26,** 139

106. Jackson, I. M. D., McKiddie, M. T. and Buchanan, K. D. (1968). The effect of prolonged fasting on carbohydrate metabolism: evidence for heterogeneity in obesity. *J. Endocrinol.,* **40,** 259

107. Suryanarayana, B. V., Kent, J. R., Meister, L. and Parlow, A. F. (1969). Pituitary-gonadal axis during prolonged total starvation in obese men. *Amer. J. Clin. Nutrition,* **22,** 767

108. Gelman, M., Sigulem, D., Sustovich, D. R., Ajzen, H. and Ramos, O. L. (1972). Starvation and renal function. *Amer. J. Med. Sci.* **263,** 465

109. Edgren, B., Wester, P. O. (1971). Impairment of glomerular filtration in fasting for obesity. *Acta Med. Scand.* **190,** 389

110. Kjellberg, J., Piscator, M., Castenfors, J. (1971). Urinary proteins and plasma renin activity during total starvation. *Acta Med. Scand.,* **190,** 519

111. Knudsen, K. B., Bradley, E. M., Lecocq., F. R., Bellamy, H. M. and Welsh, J. D. (1968). Effect of fasting and refeeding on the histology and disaccharidase activity of the human intestine. *Gastroenterology,* **55,** 46

112. Ruedi, B., Borei, G. A., Graziano, M., Frei, J. and Magnenat, P. (1969). Digestive function in obese patients during total starvation. *Schweiz. Med. Wochenschr.,* **99,** 774

113. Steiner, M., Farrish, G. C. M. and Gray, S. J. (1969). Intestinal uptake of valine in calorie and protein deprivation. *Amer. J. Clin. Nutrition,* **22,** 871

114. Adibi, S. A. and Allen, E. R. (1970). Impaired jejunal absorption rates of essential amino acids induced by either dietary caloric or protein deprivation in man. *Gastroenterology,* **59,** 404

115. Fromm, G. A., Litvak, J. and Degrossi, O. J. (1970). Intestinal absorption of calcium in fasting patients. *Lancet,* **i,** 616

116. Verdy, M. (1970). Fasting in obese females. 3. Absorption tests

(xylose, triolein, oleic acid) and cholecystography. *Amer. J. Clin. Nutrition,* **23,** 1033

117. Stanley, M. M. (1970). Quantification of intestinal functions during fasting: estimations of bile salt turnover, fecal calcium and nitrogen excretions. *Metabolism,* **19,** 865
118. Harrison, M. T. and Harden, R. McG. (1966). The long term value of fasting in the treatment of obesity. *Lancet,* **ii,** 1340
119. Hermann, L. S. and Iversen, M. (1968). Death during therapeutic starvation. *Lancet,* **ii,** 217
120. MacCuish, A. C., Munro, J. F. and Duncan, L. J. P. (1968). Follow-up study of refractory obesity treated by fasting. *Brit. Med. J.,* **i,** 91
121. Zuliani, U., Dell'Anna, A. and Cucurachi, P. (1969). Three systems of treating obesity: fasting, fasting alternated with low-energy diet, low energy diet. *Ateneo Parmense, Acta Bio-Med.,* **40,** 549
122. Coronho, V. O. (1970). Treatment of obesity by prolonged starvation. Clinical experience and review. *Rev. Assoc. Med. Minas Gerais,* **21,** 217
123. Maagøe, H. and Mogensen, E. F. (1970). The effect of treatment on obesity. A follow-up investigation of a material treated with complete starvation. *Danish Med. Bull.,* **17,** 206
124. Rooth, G. and Carleström, S. (1970). Thereapeutic fasting. *Acta Med. Scand.,* **187,** 455
125. Karns, R. M. (1966). Dramatic treatment for obesity: diseased patients test starvation diet. *J. Amer. Med. Ass.,* **197,** 22
126. Kollar, E. J., Aitkinson, R. M. and Albin, D. L. (1968). The effectiveness of fasting in the treatment of super obesity. *Psychosomatics,* **10,** 125
127. Munro, J. F., MacGuish, A. C., Wilson, E. M. and Duncan, L. J. P. (1968). Comparison of continuous and intermittent anorectic therapy in obesity. *Psychosomatics,* **11,** 352
128. Swanson, D. W. and Dinello, F. A. (1970). Follow-up of patients starved for obesity. *Psychosomatic Med.,* **32,** 209
129. Maagøe, H. (1968). Changes in blood volume during absolute fasting with and without sodium chloride administration. *Metabolism,* **17,** 133
130. Anderson, J. W., Herman, R. H. and Necomer, K. L. (1969). Improvement in glucose tolerance of fasting obese patients given oral potassium. *Amer. J. Clin. Nutrition,* **22,** 1589
131. Bittnerova, H., Rath, R. and Masek, J. (1969). Pathogenesis of

changes in water, Na and K metabolism induced by fasting in obese women. *Ces. Gastroenterol. Vyz.*, **23**, 36
132. Simeons, A. T. W. (1954). The action of Chorionic gonadotrophin in the obese. *Lancet,* **ii,** 946
133. Birkenhäger, J. C., Haak, A. and Ackers, J. G. (1968). Changes in body composition during treatment of obesity by intermittent starvation. *Metabolism,* **17,** 391
134. Pöhner, C. (1968). Treatment of obesity with a 300-kcal diet. *Ernährungs-Umschau,* **15,** 160
135. Rath, R. (1970). Relation between protein intake and N balance in obese persons in different conditions. *Ces. Gastroenterol. Vyz.,* **24,** 346
136. Matzkies, F., Baumbauer, E., Pemsel, W., Kori-Linder, C., Berg, G., Sailer, D., Grabner, W. and Bergner, D. (1972). A minimum diet in outpatient treatment of the overweight. *Medizin und Ernährung,* **13,** 97
137. Bollinger, R. E., Lukert, B. P., Brown, R. W., Guevara, L. and Steinberg, R. (1966). Metabolic balance of obese subjects during fasting. *Arch. Intern. Med.,* **118,** 3
138. Apfelbaum, M. (1968). Treatment of obesity by protein diet. *Sem. Hop. Sem. Therap.,* **44,** Th. 174-Th. 176
139. Bell, J. D., Margen, S. and Calloway, D. H. (1969). Ketosis, weight loss, uric acid, and nitrogen balance in obese women fed single nutrients at low caloric levels. *Metabolism,* **18,** 193
140. Simonyi, J., Engländer, Z., Porubszky, I., Palla, I. and Tömörkeny, M. (1969). The diuresis potentiating effect of a carbohydrate-poor diet in obese individuals and in non-obese patients with chronic congestive heart failure. *Cor Vasa,* **11,** 251
141. Katz, A. I., Hollingsworth, D. R. and Epstein, F. H. (1968). Influence of carbohydrate and protein on sodium excretion during fasting and refeeding. *J. Lab. Clin. Med.,* **72,** 93
142. Jourdan, M. H. and Bradfield, R. B. (1973). Body composition changes during weight loss estimated from energy, nitrogen, sodium and potassium balances. *Amer. J. Clin. Nutr.,* **26,** 144
143. Elsbach, P. and Schwartz, I. L. (1961). Salt and water metabolism during weight reduction. *Metabolism,* **10,** 595
144. Bloom, W. L. (1962). Inhibition of salt excretion by carbohydrate. *Arch. Intern. Med.,* **109,** 26
145. Jones, J. E., Albrink, M. J., Davidson, P. C. and Flink, E. B. (1966). Fasting and refeeding of various suboptimal isocaloric diets. *Amer. J. Clin. Nutr.,* **19,** 320

146. Russell, G. F. M. (1962). The effect of diets of different composition on weight loss, water, sodium balance in obese patients. *Clin. Sci.,* **22,** 269
147. Pilkington, T. R. E., Gainsborough, H., Rosevoer, V. M. and Carey, M. (1960). Diet and weight-reduction in the obese. *Lancet,* **i,** 856
148. Werner, S. C. (1955). Comparison between weight reduction on a high-calorie, high-fat diet and on an isocaloric regimen high in carbohydrate. *New Engl. J. Med.,* **252,** 661
149. Fletcher, R. F., McCririck, M. Y. and Crooke, A. C. (1961). Reducing diets, weight loss of obese patients on diets of different composition. *Br. J. Nutr.,* **15,** 53
150. Kinsell, L. W., Gunning, B., Michaels, G. P., Richardson, J., Cox., S. E. and Lennon, C. (1964). Calories do count. *Metabolism,* **13,** 195
151. Bortz, W. M., Wroldsen, A., Issekutz., B., and Rodahl, K. (1966). Weight loss and frequency of feeding. *New Engl. J. Med.,* **274,** 376
152. Schmidt, H., Jenik, I. and Voigt, K. D. Effects of a ketogenic diet on body-weight, intermediary and electrolyte metabolism of obese persons. *Deutsch. Med. Wochenschr.,* **94,** 78
153. Taller, H. (1962). Dietary management of obesity. *Amer. J. Obstet. Gynec.,* **83,** 62
154. Yudkin, J. and Carey, M. (1960). The treatment of obesity by the 'high-fat' diet. The inévitability of calories. *Lancet,* **ii,** 939
155. Yudkin, J. (1968). *The Complete Slimmer* (London: Macgibbon and Kee)
156. McEwen, H., Jacobson, H., Battrum, E. C., Crealock, R. J., Mitchell, M. N. and McLaren, B. A. (1972). Experience with a hospital-based weight reduction program. *Canad. Med. Ass. J.,* **107,** 43
157. Yudkin, J. (1968). Doctors' treatment of obesity. Analysis of 'The Practitioner' questionnaire. *Practitioner,* **201,** 330
158. Stock, A. L. and Yudkin, J. (1970). Nutrient intake of subjects on low carbohydrate diet used in treatment of obesity. *Amer. J. Clin. Nutrition,* **23,** 948
159. Christian, J. E., Combs, L. W. and Kessler, W. V. (1964). The body composition of obese subjects. Studies of the effect of weight loss. *Amer. J. Clin. Nutr.,* **15,** 20
160. Young, C. M. and Digiacomo, M. M. (1965). Protein utilization and changes in body composition during weight reduction. *Metabolism,* **14,** 1084

161. Bortz, W. M. A. (1969). A 500 pound weight loss. *Amer. J. Med.,* **47,** 325
162. Cederquist, D. C., Brewer, W. P., Beagle, R. M., Wagener, A. N., Dunsing, D. and Ohlson, M. A. (1952). Weight reduction on low-fat and low carbohydrate diets. *J. Amer. Diet. Ass.,* **28,** 113
163. Gordon, E. S., Goldberg, M. and Chosy, G. J. (1965). A new concept in the treatment of obesity. *J. Amer. Med. Ass.,* **186,** 50
164. Howard, A. N. and Anderson, T. B. (1968). The treatment of obesity with a high protein loaf. *Practitioner,* **201,** 491
165. Howard, A. N., Dub, I. and McMahon, M. (1971). The incidence, cause and treatment of obesity in Leicester school children. *Practitioner,* **207,** 662
166. Fabry, P., Fodor, J., Hezi, Z., Braun, T. and Zoolankova, K. (1964). The frequency of meals: its relation to overweight, hypercholesterolaemia and decreased glucose tolerance. *Lancet,* **ii,** 614
167. Rath, R., Masek, J. and Petrasek, R. (1970). Relation between the number of meals per day and body composition and some metabolic values in obese women. *Cas. Lek. Ces.,* **109,** 421
168. Bortz, W. M., Wroldsen, A., Issekutz, B. and Rodahl, K. (1966). Weight loss and frequency of feeding. *New Engl. J. Med.,* **274,** 376
169. Young, C. M., Scanlan, S. S., Topping, C. M., Simko, V. and Lutwak, L. (1971). Frequency of feeding, weight reduction, and body composition. *J. Amer. Dietet. Ass.* **59,** 466
170. Seaton, D. A. and Duncan, L. J. P. (1964). Treatment of 'Refractory Obesity' with a diet of two meals a day. *Lancet,* **ii,** 612
171. Munro, J. F., Seaton, D. A. and Duncan, L. J. P. Treatment of 'Refractory Obesity' with a diet of five meals a day. *Br. Med. J.,* **1,** 950
172. Debry, G., Rohr, R., Azouaou, G., Vassilitch, I. and Mottaz, G. (1968). Effect of dividing the daily energy intake into 7 meals on loss of weight by obese persons. *Nutritio et Dieta,* **10,** 288
173. Bloom. W. L. and Eidex, M. F. (1967). The comparison of energy expenditure in the obese and lean. *Metabolism,* **16,** 685
174. Lincoln, J. E. (1972). Calorie intake, obesity, and physical activity. *Amer. J. Clin. Nutr.,* **25,** 390
175. Bradfield, R. B., Paulos, J. and Grossman, L. (1971). Energy

expenditure and heart rate of obese high school girls. *Amer. J. Clin. Nutr.,* **24,** 1482

176. Bloom, W. L. and Eidex, M. F. (1967). Inactivity as a major factor in adult obesity. *Metabolism,* **16,** 679

177. Oscai, L. B. and Williams, B. T. (1968). Effect of exercise on overweight middle-aged males. *J. Amer. Geriat. Soc.,* **16,** 794

178. Dudleston, A. K. and Bennion, M. (1970). Effect of diet and/or exercise on obese college women. Weight loss and serum lipids. *J. Amer. Dietetic Assoc.,* **56,** 126

179. Bray, G. A., Whipp, B. J. and Koyal, S. N. (1974). The acute effects of food intake on energy expenditure during cycle ergometry. *Amer. J. Clin. Nutr.,* **27,** 254

180. Carne, S. (1961). The action of chorionic gonadotrophin in the obese. *Lancet,* **ii,** 1282

181. De Guzman, M. P. E. (1968). The group approach to weight reduction. *Philippine J. Nutrition,* **21,** 227

182. Howard, A. N. (1969). Dietary treatment of obesity. In *Obesity, Medical and Scientific Aspects.* p. 107 (Baird, I. M. and Howard, A. N., editors) (London: Livingstone)

183. Garrow, J. J. (1975). A survey of three slimming and weight control organisations in the U.K. Proc. 1st Int. Congress on Obesity (London: Newman)

6

A Behavioural Approach to the Problem of Obesity

Henry A. Jordan and
Leonard S. Levitz

Anyone who has dealt with obese patients is depressingly aware of the failure of any one treatment to lead to significant and sustained weight loss in all but a small number of cases. The difficulty and, in most cases, the failure to treat obesity effectively seems an overwhelming problem independent of the mode of therapy. Whether the treatment involves diets, drugs, starvation, psychotherapy, self-help groups, exercise programmes, or hormones, therapists have been unable to cause many persons to lose weight. In a review of the medical management of obesity, Stunkard and McLaren-Hume[1] reported that all programmes were equally ineffective in their treatment of obesity. Attrition rates in the programmes reviewed ranged from 20—80% and only 25% who stayed in therapy lost 20 lb. Furthermore, only 5% lost as much as 40 lb.

Even more disturbing than the difficulty in producing an initial weight loss are the long-term results. Of the small proportion of patients who do lose weight, almost none maintain their weight loss for more than a year. Recently, Sohar and Sneh[2] reported one of the very few long-term studies of obesity. They described the weight histories of twenty-seven obese patients who had lost an average of 28.6 lb (range 9—138 lb) during treatment fourteen years earlier. During this time, only five patients had been able to maintain their weight loss; only two patients gained in excess of 15% of their starting weight. The most surprising finding, however, was that nineteen of these twenty-seven patients weighed within 10% of what they had weighed fourteen years earlier. The long-term stability of weight found in this group of patients parallels the apparent stability of weight found among many normal weight adults, but see Chapter 1 for a fuller discussion of the question of stability of body weight.

One explanation for this long-term stability is that body weight is actually regulated in the obese individual as well as in the individual of normal weight. If this is the case, it would suggest that to formulate a successful weight reduction programme, one would need to understand the processes and determinants by which either normal or excessive body weight is regulated. No method of treating obesity can be considered without attending to these regulatory factors. It is the purpose of the present chapter to consider how a behavioural treatment approach to obesity is compatible with our present understanding of the regulation of energy balance and body weight.

REGULATION OF BODY WEIGHT

The regulation of body weight is the result of an interaction between energy intake, energy expenditure, and the net efficiency of the body's ability to convert ingested energy to expended energy (see Chapter 1). When a person maintains a stable body weight, it is assumed that a balance between energy intake and expenditure exists. It is often not recognised that an obese person, too, when maintaining a stable although elevated body weight, is maintaining a balance between intake and expenditure; hence, an equilibrium exists.

One characteristic of any biological regulatory system is a series of control mechanisms which operate to maintain equilibrium or homeostasis. When an equilibrium between energy intake and expenditure exists—regardless of the actual body weight at which it occurs—it is actively maintained by physiological and behavioural control mechanisms. If this equilibrium is disturbed and a concomitant weight change occurs, these controls operate to restore homeostasis. Therefore, any pronounced change of body weight in either direction will be difficult to maintain.

A number of studies have explored the control mechanisms which operate in the maintenance of body weight. The most detailed exploration of disturbed equilibrium in human subjects was conducted when Keys, *et al.*[3] investigated the effects of caloric restriction. Thirty-six young male volunteers were placed on an average caloric intake of 1570 kcal/day for six months. This level was considerably below maintenance. The most obvious effect was an expected weight loss—subjects had an average decrease of 24% body weight. However, in addition to weight loss, the following effects of the disturbance of energy equilibrium were noted: (*a*) pulse rate dropped; (*b*) basal metabolic rate dropped; (*c*) general activity slowed down; (*d*) libido decreased; (*e*) tolerance to heat increased; (*f*) tolerance to cold decreased; and (*g*) vertigo and giddiness occurred. The first four observations reflect physiological and metabolic alterations which in one way or another are evidence of the organism's attempt to restore energy balance through the conservation of energy. Since the subjects were unable to increase their intake of energy, the last three changes and their weight losses reflect the organism's failure to maintain equilibrium.

In addition to these effects, other changes were observed which reflected the subjects' increased desire for food. Anticipation of eating became exaggerated, craving for and preoccupation with food increased, dislikes for certain foods disappeared, and socially acceptable eating behaviour such as table manners disintegrated. In addition, depression, apathy, and general irritability increased. It is noteworthy that when food intake was no longer restricted, these changes in behaviour and emotion persisted for several months. From this study it is apparent that humans have physiological and behavioural control systems which serve as protection against energy deficits.

It is equally important to determine whether there are similar controls which operate to protect man from the intake and storage of excess energy. In other words, does excessive food intake in a thin or normal weight individual lead to obesity, or are there mechanisms for resisting or slowing weight gain? Studies investigating this question are not nearly as numerous as those concerned with caloric restriction, but there have been a few attempts to produce experimental obesity in man.

Sims and co-workers at the University of Vermont attempted to induce excessive weight gain in four normal-weight college students by having them ingest two or three times their normal caloric intake each day for three to five months[4]. In this investigation, it soon became apparent that increasing the weight of these individuals was as difficult as decreasing weight in subjects in starvation studies. At the end of the experimental period, the weight gain was 10—12% of the starting weight. If this rate of gain had been sustained, a marked degree of obesity would have occurred after two or three years, but there was evidence during this forced feeding period that controls were operating to resist excessive weight gain. For instance, subjects became more reluctant to eat. More important, the degree of weight gain expected from the surplus number of calories ingested often did not occur. Repeating the study under more controlled circumstances (with nine inmates of a prison), a 26% increase in body weight occurred, double the amount gained and at twice the rate as in the earlier study. However, even in the prison study, some subjects were more resistant to weight gain than others. Although the reasons for this are not clearly understood, it was apparent that the inmates' level of spontaneous activity was an important factor. Weight increased most rapidly in those individuals whose spontaneous activity appeared low. The most striking finding of this study was that when forced feeding was terminated, weights rapidly returned to pre-experimental levels.

In a similar vein, Miller and Mumford conducted experiments[5] in which sixteen normal-weight subjects received an average of 1400 kcal/day above their usual intake for four to eight weeks. They were given either high- or low-protein diets, and weights and metabolic rates were determined for all subjects. The weight gain expected from the excessive calories did not occur. In fact, a subject receiving an excess of 8000—10 000 kcal/week occasionally lost weight. The most weight gained by any subject during the eight-week period was 10 lb, an increase of 7% of initial body weight. The authors concluded that, in the face of excess input of calories, metabolic changes occurred which increased subjects' expenditure of energy. Thus weight gain was resisted.

Quite clearly, then, the individual of normal weight resists alterations in energy balance in either a positive or negative direction and defends a stable body weight[6].

One of the reasons for the inability of the obese individual to maintain a reduced body weight may be that he is below a set point of equilibrium. If this is the case, then one would expect effects similar to those found among the volunteers in the study by Keys and Brozek. There are a number of studies which have investigated the psychological, behavioural, and physiological response of obese individuals to caloric restriction and weight loss. For example, several investigators[7,8] report that there are numerous untoward reactions to caloric restriction in obese patients. They become irritable, preoccupied with food, and in many instances depressed. Furthermore, Bray[9] has reported that metabolic rate decreased when obese subjects were placed on a rigid regimen of 450 calories/day. These subjects' metabolic rates had an average decrease of 15% as measured by oxygen consumption. As a result of this reduced metabolic rate their weight loss did not equal that expected from such a degree of caloric restriction. It appears, then, that the obese person may be just as resistant to weight loss as the normal weight person, and when placed on a restricted diet may suffer just as much as a normal weight person.

THE DETERMINANTS OF FOOD INTAKE

All therapeutic regimens for obesity must necessarily create a disequilibrium in energy balance. Because the organism will strive to return to equilibrium, any method of weight reduction which does not cause a permanent change in energy intake or expenditure, or in the organism's biological make-up, will not result in long-term maintenance of altered body weight. In order to achieve such changes, it is necessary to alter one or another of the essential determinants governing the equilibrium between energy intake and expenditure.

We have found it helpful to organise the determinants of energy intake into a multistage schema, shown in Figure 6.1. The first stage is composed of biological processes which may be genetic, anatomical, physiological, and/or biochemical in nature. The result of these biological processes are then modulated by two different sets of environmental and experiential factors. The result of these modulations produce the specific behaviours which are involved in an organism's initiation of eating, selection of food, and termination of food intake. Once these three behaviours are known, one can account for an organism's total food intake in any given period of time. The specific variables listed in Figure 6.1 represent only a subset of the possible factors influencing food intake, and as such are to be taken as examples, but the types of essential determinants illustrated operate in the control of ingestion in both normal weight and obese organisms.

In and of itself, the set of biological processes involved in the control of food intake is immensely complex. These determinants, which have a primary genetic basis, tend to be stable over long periods of time and are more immutable than the factors subsumed under Modulations I and II. The biological factors determine the impact of the modulating factors upon eating behaviour. For example, a profound energy deficit produced by starvation may have a direct influence upon the type of food selected and volume of food ingested regardless of such factors as the food's palatability or cost, or the physical circumstances under which ingestion occurs. As was shown by Keys *et al.*[3], during semi-starvation, prior food dislikes disappear, rates of ingestion are altered, and social amenities usually associated with eating change.

While it is not feasible in this chapter to review the immense amount of work that has helped detail the effect of biological processes upon ingestion, it must be kept in mind that they are of primary importance in accounting for the behaviours involved in energy regulation. However, in almost all cases, these biological processes are influenced by, and interact with, other determinants involved in food intake.

At one level, the result of biological processes are modulated by a number of psychological, cultural, and familial factors. These factors also tend to be stable over long periods of time, but unlike the biological

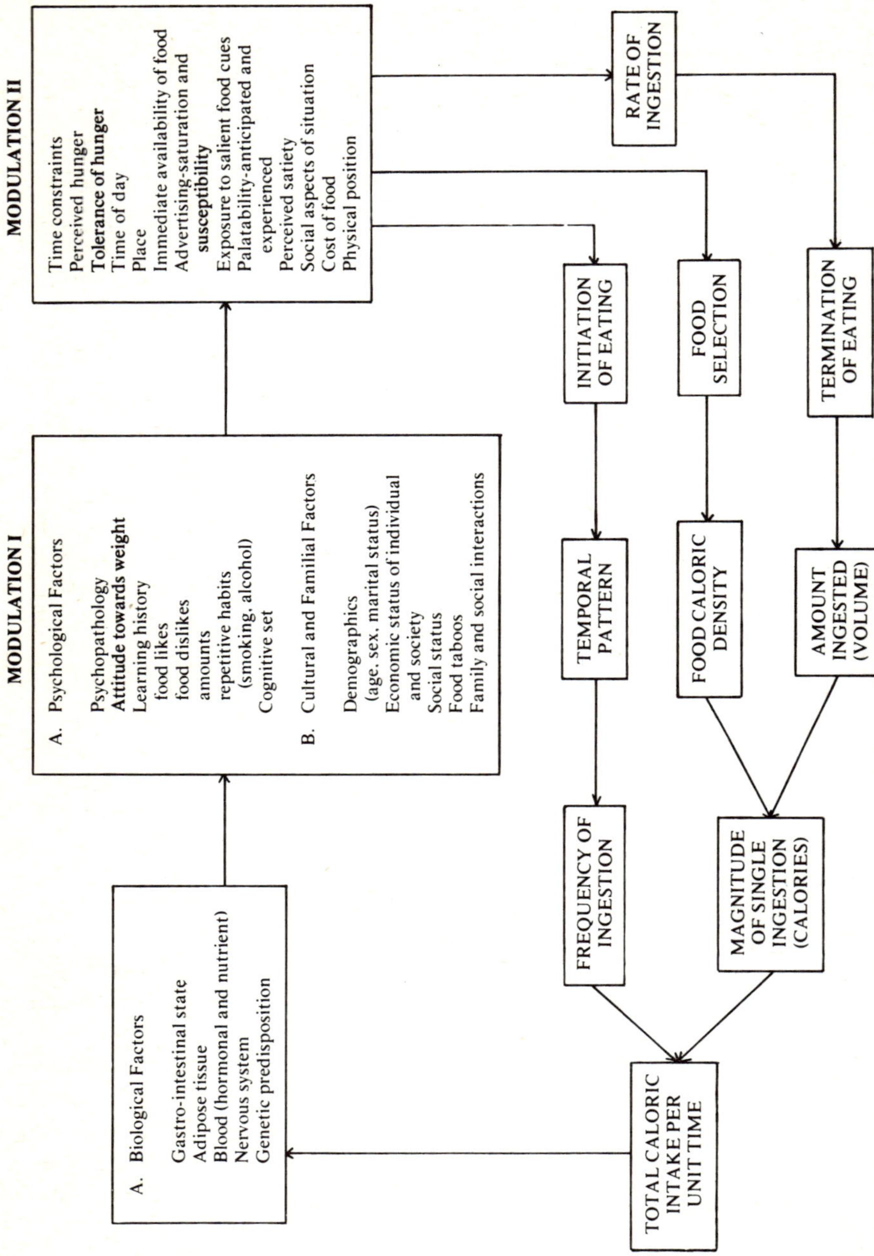

FIGURE 6.1 The determinants of food intake

factors, most of these are primarily determined by the individual's early experiences with his environment. For example, early disturbances of psychological processes[10], as well as normal socialisation processes may determine early food preferences which then play a role in determining a person's life-long selection of foods.

Similarly, food selections are strongly influenced by broad cultural factors such as food taboos and the overall availability of particular foods in the society. The social and economic status of the individual and his family may also account for the type and amount of food generally available for consumption.

In every family, early learning experiences shape patterns of behaviour which tend to be stable throughout a person's life. As each child has different genetic and environmental influences, so he develops different behaviours which enter into the regulation of energy balance and weight.

If one observes the eating behaviour of a newborn infant, it is easily seen how parental teaching and attitudes begin to influence these behaviours. For example, the breast-fed child sucks until satisfied and the mother does not know how much milk he has ingested. Physiologically, however, the mother produces milk according to the demands of the child. This important biological feedback system is completely disrupted when the breast is replaced by a bottle. Now the mother has a visual cue and can see how much milk the child has ingested. She can now use this cue to shape a child's eating behaviour according to her own attitudes about how much the child should eat. It now becomes possible for her to over- or underfeed her child. Beginning with this process, the parent assumes a much greater role in teaching, shaping and modeling feeding behaviour.

In most instances, these learned behaviours result in the regulation of normal body weight. However, Ullmann[11] has outlined a number of ways by which a child may develop inappropriate eating habit patterns which lead to disorders in energy balance. First, the child may learn to depend on environmental cues for the termination of food intake. In the previous example of breast versus bottle feeding, the relationship between food delivery and the child's physiological needs is disrupted. As this occurs a child may be taught to rely on the cues provided by the parent rather than those provided by his own physiological needs. A common example of this process is when parental approval is given or withheld in association with the amount of food remaining on the child's plate. Through repetition of this process, the cue for meal termination is no longer an internal satiety signal but becomes the act of 'cleaning the plate'. In addition, food itself is a strong 'positive reinforcer' as it satisfies physiological needs. Therefore, food may come to satisfy multiple emotional needs by being strongly and repeatedly associated with parental attention, comfort and affection. Through this association, food may become a general way of coping with various emotional states. For instance, food can be used to reduce anxiety, alleviate pain, lift depression, relieve boredom, distract from loneliness, counter fatigue or even enhance happiness.

Eating occurs in many situations and under a variety of conditions and experiences, and therefore ingestive behaviour may come to be controlled by many influences other than those based on biological processes. Not only may parents actively teach inappropriate early eating behaviours and uses for food, but because the child patterns much of his behaviour after that of his parents, the eating behaviours of the parent become incorporated into the repertoire of the child. It is through such behavioural developments as these that learning processes enter into the regulation of energy balance.

The result of these psychological, cultural and familial determinants are further modulated by factors which are present in the immediate environment and perception of the individual. By varying greatly from one individual to another, these factors lead to important differences in the behaviours occurring immediately before, during and after ingestion. Each person, because of repeated experience with these Modulation II factors, develops stable associations between the immediate factors and the behaviours involved in food intake. For example, infants do not eat three meals a day. Through maturation of the biological system, together with socialisation processes in the family, and through cues in the immediate environment, this temporal pattern of eating most often develops in our society. This pattern, in fact, may become so overlearned that even though a person could biologically afford to skip a meal, he will not do so if the appropriate cues previously associated with eating are present in the immediate environment. He will eat without necessarily being in a state of energy deficit. On the other hand, if the cues are not present, he may not eat even if he is in a state of energy deficit.

The interaction of biological factors with Modulation I and II factors determine the probability of food intake being initiated, and the probability of a particular food being selected. The probability of food intake being terminated at a given time depends on these same factors, but in interaction with the rate of ingestion.

Once we understand the determinants influencing the initiation and termination of ingestion and food selection, we can then account for the magnitude and frequency of each eating event and the total caloric intake in a given period of time.

Although we will not present a model of the determinants of energy expenditure, the same types of determinants are involved. These determinants influence three parameters of activity; namely, the frequency, duration, and type of energy expenditure.

While not shown in Figure 6.1 for the sake of simplicity, it must be recognised that interactions between all determinants occur. The most apt description of the complexity of energy regulation was brought into the literature on eating behaviour by Hilde Bruch[10] when she quoted the naturalist John Muir: 'When we try to pick out anything by itself, we usually find it hitched to everything else in the universe.'

TREATMENT MODALITIES

The schema presented here helps to categorise the way in which various treatment modalities attempt to alter food intake. A cure for obesity has been known for centuries. For example, Brillat-Savarin[12] in 1825 states: 'Any cure for obesity must begin with the three following and absolute precepts: discretion in eating, moderation in sleeping, and exercise on foot and horseback.' In other words, decrease food intake and increase physical activity. But this 'cure' focuses only on the outcome of all the determinants involved in energy regulation. Similarly, by simply advising a patient to decrease the frequency of ingestive events by cutting out snacks and to decrease the magnitude of ingestion by eating less at each meal, we provide him with no tools or guidelines with which to accomplish this outcome. It is not surprising, then, that this approach most commonly fails.

Hospital starvation programmes which decrease the frequency and magnitude of eating to zero and achieve rapid weight loss also do not change the essential determinants of food intake. One would expect that when the individual returns to his usual environment and is once again exposed to the Modulation I and II factors, he will return to former behaviour patterns and regain weight.

Another treatment approach prescribes specific foods, amounts, and temporal patterns. Most dietary approaches operate at this level (see Chapter 5). A person is told what to eat, how much to eat, and when to eat. Although some diets prescribe all three, most often limits are set on only one or two of these parameters. These programmes, too, will succeed so long as the person is able to adhere strictly to the prescribed guidelines. But what usually happens is that most patients are unable to continue with these guidelines for more than a short period of time because they are continually exposed to the unchanged determinants of their previous eating patterns. In addition to regaining weight, the patient has the added frustration of knowing he has failed.

A number of drug and hormonal therapies have been directed at altering the basic biological factors determining food intake (see Chapter 7). This is a traditional site of successful intervention in many disease states. But the problem in obesity is that no treatment procedure has been shown to change the biological processes effectively over a long period of time. The bowel bypass procedure produces a biological change that actually nullifies the end result of all other determinants by not allowing most of the ingested calories to be utilised. This drastic procedure, however, is often accompanied by serious complications and cannot be regarded as a preferred treatment for most cases of obesity.

Traditional psychotherapy is clearly aimed at producing changes in the psychological factors included under Modulation I. In cases where it can be determined that primary psychopathology is a major determinant of overeating, this treatment approach would be indicated. However, in the overwhelming majority of cases any psychopathology observed is secondary or coincidental to the development of obesity.

Many programmes have been suggested which operate at the cultural and familial level for the prevention and treatment of obesity. For example, national education programmes and food engineering proposals are aimed at promoting alterations in cultural habits, biases and overall food supplies. It has also been suggested from the work of Hirsch and Knittle[13] that early changes in infant nutrition to prevent overfeeding may constrain fat cell number and thus help to prevent the development of obesity. However, at the present time, such constraints must be produced by changes in Modulation I and II factors.

Currently, then, we must recognise the necessity for changing some of the essential determinants of food intake; but we must also recognise that promoting changes in the biological determinants and broad social and cultural determinants are not presently feasible. What seems indicated is a programme in which we attempt to alter the susceptibility, exposure, and response of a patient to those Modulation I and II factors which influence his maladaptive feeding behaviour. Appropriate alterations in response to these essential determinants will produce adaptive changes in eating behaviour and activity patterns and hence weight loss. The locus of control, from the outset, must be with the patient so that response changes to the Modulation I and II factors will persist and thus reduce the probability that weight lost will be regained.

BEHAVIOUR MODIFICATION

During the past two decades a variety of techniques based upon learning theory and aimed at the modification of human behaviour have been devised and evaluated (see Appendix 1 for full bibliography). The major techniques which have been applied to the problem of obesity fall into four broad classifications:

(1) *Aversive control*—in which a real or imagined aversive stimulus (nausea, electric shock) is associated with a favourite food or with a cognitive representation of eating behaviour.

(2) *Contingency management*—in which specific positive or negative consequences are attached to desirable or undesirable eating behaviours or weight changes. The contingency between the behaviour and its consequence may be managed (administered) by either the patient or by the therapist.

(3) *Environmental management*—in which the patient is instructed in specific ways to change his environment so as to increase the probability of adaptive eating behaviour.

(4) *Self-monitoring*—of either eating behaviour or weight change, by which the person keeps a continuous record of his behaviours, their antecedents, and their consequences.

Recently a number of excellent reviews (Abramson[14], Hall and Hall[15], Stuart[16], Stunkard[17]) of this rapidly growing literature have been prepared, and although no attempt will be made to re-evaluate the findings of the fifty-three case studies and experimental investigations listed in the appendix of this chapter the conclusions drawn by several of the authors are as follow.

Stunkard[17] concluded that 'both greater loss during treatment and superior maintenance of weight loss after treatment indicated that behaviour modification is more effective than previous methods of treatment for obesity'. Stuart[16] states that behaviour modification techniques are at the moment the most promising approach to the management of overeating and underexercising. However, he cautions against generalised optimism before the long range effectiveness for various types of obesity are known. Hall and Hall[15] also state that the techniques are promising but that further work will be required to refine the technology.

Most of the recent studies have concentrated on the effects of self-monitoring, contingency management and environmental control. As Abramson stated in his review, 'It appears safe to conclude that despite some early enthusiasm, there is little evidence to indicate that aversive procedures are an effective treatment for obesity. The reported outcomes of the case studies are equivocal at best'[14].

The large number of studies which can be cited in this area of research should not be interpreted as a sign that behaviour modification has found a complete answer to the problem of obesity. At the present time the greatest need in this area is the collection of long-term follow-up data. The studies do indicate, however, that behaviour modification for obesity is an active field which is continuing to explore a variety of psychological techniques with which promising results have been demonstrated.

In a behavioural approach the focus of attention is on observable behaviour and observed behaviour change. The therapist and patient are most interested in the specific behaviours that should be increased, decreased, eliminated, or instituted.

The most distinctive characteristic of behaviour therapy is that it attempts to abstract effective clinical techniques from general psychological principles, primarily from research in human learning and social psychology. For example, independent of the specific technique, a process of *shaping* is implied throughout the therapeutic programme. Shaping refers to a process of providing for small, incremental changes in a behaviour, with each step more closely approximating the final goal behaviour. If eating a particular high-caloric food represents a major habit problem, the final goal — to reach a low level of consumption—would be gradually approached in a series of discrete steps. In working with the overweight person, this principle is also applied to the progression of weight loss. A gradual weight loss of from 1—2 lb/week is generally stated as the criterion for successful progress[18].

In several respects, overeating is one of the most complex behaviour problems that has been approached by behaviour therapy. Not only has it proved very resistant to most types of therapeutic intervention, but the physiological limitations on any intervention are not known. Moreover, treatment is complex because it must rely on principles of self-management, which means that the processes of behaviour-monitoring and behaviour change are under the control of the patient. (In many other areas, the same techniques of behaviour change have been administered by outside agents—psychotherapists, teachers, psychiatric nurses, or hospital aides.) While there is evidence that self-management can effect behaviour changes as profound as those achieved by externally administered treatment[19] there are many questions about self-management that still must be researched[20].

When the success of treatment depends on self-management, the purpose of therapeutic contacts is to provide the patient with techniques for achieving appropriate behaviour changes. In the treatment of obesity, an educational approach is taken in which a principal role of the therapist is to teach the patient how to analyse his own behaviour patterns and how to devise suitable techniques for changing them.

Thus, behaviour therapy, as applied to obesity, is characterised by:

(*a*) determination of observable eating and activity habit patterns; (*b*) measurement of the target behaviours before and during treatment; (*c*) a series of techniques abstracted from psychological research in learning; and (*d*) an educational approach to the development of self-management.

In most disease states, whether physiological or psychological, we consider the problem to be a result of some abnormal functioning of the organism. For example, in heart disease one talks of abnormalities in heart structure and function, in mental retardation about abnormalities in central nervous system structure and function. In disorders of energy balance, however, there is no clear distinction between normal and abnormal eating behaviour or normal and abnormal activity patterns. Therefore, rather than label these behaviours as normal or abnormal we must consider to what extent each particular behaviour contributes to either an appropriate or an inappropriate level of stored adipose tissue.

In the treatment of obesity, those behaviours which contribute to a high intake of calories or a low expenditure of energy are viewed as inappropriate and maladaptive. For example, eating nuts or popcorn while watching TV (high caloric input—low expenditure of energy) is not maladaptive for a thin person but is clearly maladaptive for an obese person who is actually gaining weight or is attempting to lose weight. The same can be said for the rapid ingestion of a piece of cheesecake while standing in front of the refrigerator. In a similar fashion the amount of time a person spends either sitting down or lying down may be adaptive or maladaptive depending on the weight and goals of the individual. For example, the total reliance on the automobile as a means of locomotion constitutes no problem and is adaptive from an energy efficiency standpoint for the normal weight person. But for an obese individual who is attempting to create a negative energy balance, this conservation of expended energy is clearly contrary to his goals.

As in any treatment programme for obesity, the first step is to gain an understanding of the biological, psychological and cultural factors which pertain to each individual obese patient. The following information is required:

1. Weight history (age of onset, peak weight, previous weight loss attempts and successes)
2. Psychological evaluation (by interview and psychological testing)
3. Medical history
4. Family history of obesity and related disorders
5. Socioeconomic and cultural factors and demographics.

This information is necessary to assess the contribution of the biological and Modulation I factors to the control of food intake and energy expenditure.

The next step in a behaviour modification programme is a functional analysis of the patient's eating behaviour. The purpose of this analysis is to describe (*a*) the type of habit patterns and their frequencies or rates of occurrence, and (*b*) the determinants of these habit patterns. In order to evaluate the effect of any given determinant upon either the initiation, selection, rate or termination of eating, patients are taught to monitor their own feeding behaviours. The record kept by the patient should include the frequency, duration and magnitude of the target behaviours together with some of the potentially important Modulation II determinants. Recording is done continuously by the patient for each and every incidence of ingestion, and the following information is recorded for each ingestive event:

1. Time of initiation of eating;
2. Time of termination of eating;
3. Place of eating;
4. Physical position of eating;
5. Social aspects of the situation;
6. Activities associated with eating;
7. Perceived degree of hunger;
8. Perceived mood;
9. Food selected;
10. Amount consumed—by volume and by calories.

In addition to recording the parameters involved in feeding behaviour, patients also record two parameters of energy expenditure: (1) the level of energy expenditure as indicated by the type of physical activity and (2) the place where the activity occurs (see Appendix 2).

During the first week of record keeping, patients are instructed to try and maintain their usual eating and activity patterns. However, an initial reduction in food intake as a result of the self-monitoring procedure alone is frequently noted[20]. Most often, the nature of this change appears to be in the area of food selections. However, the associations between the determinants monitored and ingestive behaviour are still evident.

Following the completion of these records it is absolutely imperative that those behaviours which can be considered maladaptive are correctly identified. This is an essential task because a behaviour which is maladaptive for one obese person may not be maladaptive for another. For instance, it has been suggested that the rate of eating is related to the amount of food ingested. While rapid eating may or may not be a habit that differentiates obese from normal weight individuals, for some obese people this habit may account for a large part of overeating and thus is maladaptive. For other obese patients, however, a fast pace of eating may contribute only minimally to the problem of overeating.

Incorrect assessment of the behaviours that are truly maladaptive for each patient will lead during treatment to random behavioural change. This will only serve to frustrate further both patient and therapist. Alteration of long-standing habits is difficult, and changing behaviours which do not contribute significantly to the disordered energy balance will not lead to weight loss.

Because this is such an important step in this treatment approach, a precise method of analysis is necessary. Simply scanning the food intake records to arrive at a clinical judgment of problem areas does not provide the precision required for a proper diagnosis.

In the functional analysis, one must determine the effect each factor has on the behaviours involved in food selection, initiation, termination, and rate. We have devised a method of analysis by which one can summarise the frequency of ingestion (initiation), rate of ingestion, amount consumed and food selection associated with each of the Modulation II factors sampled on the food intake record. The analysis indicates those areas which are not in keeping with the creation of a negative energy balance and hence weight loss.

From this analysis, for example, one might note that a high frequency of ingestions is occurring while the patient is alone. One would then look again at the food record specifically for those instances when the patient is eating alone. If the caloric value (amount and/or caloric density) of the food ingested while alone is high we conclude that eating alone is maladaptive for the patient. We have seen situations where this has been dramatically underscored: not only has caloric intake been high when ingestions occurred while the patient was eating alone, but intake was low when he was eating with others. This method of analysis is used for each determinant of ingestion so that the end result is a set of eating habits, each of which is either adaptive or maladaptive to the patient's goal of losing weight or maintaining weight loss. It is important to note interactions among parameters in order to specify the maladaptive habits precisely.

It is often stated that obese persons select inappropriate foods which are of high caloric density and poor nutritional content. When this is the case it is not enough to simply tell the person to eat different foods. It is essential to identify the determinants associated with these food selections. By means of this analysis one is then in a position to alter food selections.

Once the entire cluster of determinants surrounding the maladaptive behaviours have been identified, specific recommendations and techniques for altering the maladaptive habits can be suggested to the patient. Although there are only a few general laws of learning, numerous therapeutic techniques can be derived from them. Selection of a particular technique must be based on the initial behavioural analysis so that there is a clear correspondence between the maladaptive habit and the technique chosen to effect the change.

Behaviour change is often seen as an all-or-none affair: a person either eats dessert or he does not eat dessert. As mentioned previously, the general principle of learning is that behaviour change proceeds most effectively by means of a series of small incremental changes, each step more closely approximating the final goal. From this general principle many specific techniques may be derived. While the same underlying principles of learning can be employed, the specific content and order of the programme must be defined by the results of the original functional analysis.

Using a behaviour mentioned previously, an obese individual may habitually consume all the food on his plate regardless of the amount placed before him. The patient is using a clean plate as the signal for meal termination rather than a signal based on some internal physiological satiety mechanism. The ultimate behavioural goal in reversing this maladaptive habit is to change the signal that indicates the end of the meal. It is unrealistic to expect the patient to change this long practiced and automatic behaviour overnight. Therefore, one utilises the principle of shaping to devise a series of steps leading to the ultimate goal. The steps are programmed according to the patient's progress and designed to afford a high probability of success at each phase. The first step might be to leave over one teaspoon of food at the dinner meal. The frequency of the response and the amount remaining can then be increased over a period of time.

During the course of treatment a series of techniques for changing the identified maladaptive habits are suggested. The patient's food record may indicate a problem in the act of ingestion such as eating too fast, taking large bites, or being generally unaware of amounts consumed. Techniques would be directed at teaching the patient to pause between bites, cut food into smaller pieces, delay between courses, and concentrate on the sight, smell, and taste of the food. The records may also show that eating occurs in connection with a wide variety of stimuli such as a particular time of day, being in a particular place, or being in the presence of food. The patient should learn to confine his eating to a narrow range of stimuli. For example, he would gradually restrict eating to only certain times of the day, to one room of the house, and reduce visible food supplies through altered shopping, storage and preparation habits. If the analysis shows that activities occurring during ingestion such as watching television or reading are instrumental in producing inappropriate eating behaviour, then the patient is instructed to make eating a singular experience.

In many cases, emotional states such as boredom, depression, or anxiety, serve as determinants for maladaptive eating behaviour. While it is sometimes necessary clinically to treat the patient's response to the antecedent conditions producing the emotional state, it may be that he has learned to use food as a means of relieving mild anxiety or boredom. In such cases, it is not the emotional reaction that differentiates the obese from the normal-weight person, but rather his response to it. This association between an emotional antecedent and eating can be viewed as a learned maladaptive habit that is susceptible to behavioural change.

During treatment, the concept of programming incompatible behaviours is useful in altering this type of habit. An incompatible behaviour should be one which (*a*) the patient finds enjoyable, (*b*) is readily available, and (*c*) cannot be engaged in while eating. Ideally, it should also be an activity which promotes energy expenditure. Patients are instructed to use such activities as alternatives to eating when they find themselves bored, mildly depressed, or anxious.

The idea of 'doing something other than eating' can be extended to include alternative activities that are not necessarily incompatible with eating, giving the patient a wider choice of activities. Errands, hobbies, reading, and work activities can be planned for the times of day when he is most likely to experience negative affect states. Often a project list of short-term household or work activities provides readily available alternatives to eating in response to a particular feeling.

Another set of problem habits is often found in the temporal pattern of ingestion. In one case, there may be no pattern at all: food is likely to be consumed during any waking hour. On the other hand, there may be one particular time during the day when high caloric foods are consumed. For some patients, an effective technique is to carefully pre-plan the day's food intake early in the morning. Essentially, the person completes the food record prior to ingestion and writes down beforehand what foods, in what amounts, and at what times he will eat. In one experimental study[21] pre-recording was shown to exert more control over food intake than post-recording.

For most individuals, the temporal pattern of ingestion reflects their general lifestyle and routine. Frequently, it is necessary to recommend changes in the patient's daily routines so as to decrease exposure to food, to boredom, to time constraints during mealtimes or to stress just prior to ingestion.

After the patient is instructed in a behavioural technique, the record keeping and analysis provide week to week feedback on changes he has accomplished in the target habits. By the use of behaviour recording and analysis the patient is able to set realistic goals for stepwise changes of behaviour and then to observe his progress towards his goals.

In a similar fashion one can devise techniques for increasing physical activity, which is as important as altering feeding behaviours in producing a negative energy balance. An obese and sedentary person will not be able to go out and run a mile or play a set of tennis; this would represent not only a physiological stress but an abrupt and major behavioural change. A more logical approach is to identify those activities in which the patient currently engages and gradually to increase the frequency, intensity and duration of these activities. For example, the frequency, intensity, and duration of walking may be increased by any one of the following: (1) parking one's car further from one's destination; (2) walking more briskly; (3) walking short distances instead of using meachnical transportation; or (4) using stairs in place of elevators and escalators. All these changes, like those surrounding eating, can be accomplished in gradual steps.

The behavioural treatment programme, then, is composed of a wide variety of techniques, each providing a partial solution to the maladaptive habits of the obese patient. Repetition of habit changes which are incorporated into the daily routine and lifestyle of the patient and seen by him to be directly related to weight loss enhance long-term success. Through this process of daily record keeping, weekly analysis, and slow behaviour change in both eating behaviour and physical activity, the patient assumes responsibility for his own behaviour, which must remain the ultimate goal of the treatment programme.

Appendix 1

Bibliography of Behaviour Therapy in Obesity

Key: Aversive Control A; Contingency Management B; Environmental Management C; Self Monitoring D.

1962

1. Ferster, C. B., Nurnberger, J. T. and Levitt, E. B. The control of eating *J. Mathetics,* **1,** 87 C, D

1963

2. Allyon, T. Intensive treatment of psychotic behavior by stimulus satiation and food reinforcement. *Behar. Res. Ther.,* **1,** 53 B

1964

3. Meyer, V. and Crisp, A. H. Aversion therapy in two cases of obesity. *Behav. Res. Ther.,* **2,** 143 A
4. Thorpe, J. G., Schmidt, E., Brown, P. T. and Castell, D. Aversion-relief therapy: a new method for general application. *Behav. Res. Ther.,* **2,** 71 A

1965

5. Goldiamond, I. Self-control procedures in personal behaviour problems. *Psychol. Rep.,* **17,** 861 B, C

1966

6. Cautela, J. R. Treatment of compulsive behaviour by covert sensitization. *Psychol. Rec.,* **16,** 33 A, D

1967

7. Stollack, G. E. Weight loss obtained under different experimental procedures. *Psychother. Theor. Res. Pract.*, **6,** 61 A, D
8. Stuart, R. B. Behavioral control of overeating. *Behav. Res. Ther.*, **5,** 357 A, B, C, D

1968

9. Bernard, J. L. Rapid treatment of gross obesity by operant techniques. *Psychol. Rep.*, **23,** 663 B
10. Harmatz, M. G. and Lapuc, P. Behavior modification of overeating in a psychiatric population. *J. Consult. Clin. Psychol,* **32,** 583 B
11. Kennedy, W. A. and Foreyt, J. Control of eating behavior in an obese patient by avoidance conditioning. *Psychol. Rep.*, **22,** 571 A

1969

12. Harris, M. Self-directed program for weight control. *J. Abn. Psychol.*, **74,** 263 A, C, D
13. Moore, C. W. and Crum, B. C. Weight reduction in a chronic schizophrenic by means of operant conditioning procedures: a case study. *Behav. Res. Ther.*, **7,** 129 B

1970

14. Meynen, G. E. A comparative study of three treatment approaches with the obese: relaxation, covert sensitization and modified systematic densensitization. *Diss. Abstr. Int.* **31** (5-B), 2998 A
15. Tyler, V. O. and Straughan, J. H. Coverant control and breath holding as techniques for the treatment of obesity. *Psychol. Rec.*, **20,** 473 A
16. Wollersheim, J. P. Effectiveness of group therapy based upon learning principles in the treatment of overweight women. *J. Abn. Psychol.*, **76,** 462 B, C

16a. Shipman, W. Behavior therapy with obese dieters. Annual report of the Institute for Psychosomatic and Psychiatric Research and Training, Michael Reese Hospital and Medical Center, Chicago, p. 70 B, C

1971

17. Harris, M. and Bruner, C. G. A comparison of a self-control and a contract procedure for weight control. *Behav. Res. Ther.*, **9,** 347 B, C, D

18. Foreyt, J. P. and Kennedy, W. A. Treatment of overweight by aversion therapy. *Behav. Res. Ther.*, **9,** 29 A, D
19. Horan, J. J. and Johnson, R. G. Coverant conditioning through a self-management application of the Premack principle: its effect on weight reduction. *J. Behav. Ther. Exper. Psychiat.*, **2**, 243 A, B
20. Stuart, R. B. A three dimensional program for the treatment of obesity. *Beh. Res. Ther.*, **9,** 177 C,D
21. Upper, D. and Newton, J. G. A weight reduction program for schizophrenic patients on a token economy unit: two case studies. *J. Behav. Ther. Exper. Psychiat.*, **2,** 113 B

1972

22. Deitchman, P. The use of covert sensitization in the treatment of obesity. (Unpub. doct. diss., Florida St. Univ.) A
23. Dinoff, M., Richard, H. C. and Colwick, J. Weight reduction through successive contracts. *Amer. J. Orthopsychiat.*, **42,** 110 B
24. Haffey, V., Soroko, M. and McCormack, J. Use of modeling and of operant reinforcement procedures in a group weight reduction program. *Newsl. Res. Psychol.*, **14,** 17
25. Hall, S. M. Self-control and therapist control in the behavioral treatment of overweight women. *Behav. Res. Ther.*, **10**, 59 B, C, D
26. Janda, L. H. and Rimm, D. C. Covert sensitization in the treatment of obesity. *J. Abn. Psychol.*, **80,** 37 A
27. Jeffrey, D. B. and Christensen, E. R. The relative efficacy of behavior therapy, will power and no-treatment control procedures for weight loss. Paper read at Assn. Adv. Behav. Ther. meeting, New York City. B, C, D
28. Jeffrey, D. B., Christensen, E. R. and Pappas, J. P. A case study report of a behaviour modification weight reduction group: treatment and follow-up. *Res. Devel. Rep.*, **33,** Univ Utah Counseling Center B, D
29. Korman, I. B. The effectiveness of contractual management in weight reduction groups. (Unpub. doct. diss, Univ. Oregon) B
30. Mann, R. A. The behavior therapeutic use of contingency contracting to control an adult behavior problem: weight control. *J. Appl. Behav. Anal.*, **5,** 99 B
31. Manno, E. B. Weight reduction as a function of the timing of reinforcement in a covert aversive conditioning paradigm. *Diss. Abstr. Int.*, **32** (7-B) 4221 A
32. Manno, B. and Marston, A. R. Weight reduction as a function of

negative covert reinforcement (sensitization) versus positive covert reinforcement. *Behav. Res. Ther.*, **10**, 201 A, C, D

33. Murray, D. C. and Harrington, L. G. Covert aversive sensitization in the treatment of obesity. *Psychol. Rep.*, **30**, 560 A
34. Penick, S., Filion, R., Fox, S. and Stunkard, A. J. Behavior modification in the treatment of obesity. *Psychosom. Med.*, **33**, 49 C, D
35. Sachs, L. B. and Ingram, G. L. Covert sensitization as a treatment for weight control.*Psychol. Rep.*, **30**, 971 A
36. Shipley, L. L. and Frey, M. Two approaches to weight control. *Rehab. Psychol.*, **19**, 169 D
37. Tobias, L. L. The relative effectiveness of behavioristic bibliotherapy, contingency contracting and suggestions of self-control in weight reduction. (Unpub. doct. diss, Univ. Illinois) B, C

1973

38. Bornstein, P. H. and Sipprelle, C. N. Induced anxiety in the treatment of obesity: a preliminary case report. *Behav. Ther.*, **4**, 141 A
39. Bornstein, P. H. and Sipprelle, C. N. Group treatment of obesity by induced anxiety. *Behav. Res. Ther.*, **11**, 339 A
40. Foreyt, J. P., Hagen, R. L. Covert sensitization: conditioning or suggestion. *J. Abnormal. Psychol.*, **82**, 17 A
41. Fowler, R. S. Fordyce, W. E., Boyd, V. D. and Masock, A. J. The mouthful diet: a behavioral approach to overeating. *Rehab. Psychol.*, **19**, 98
42. Hall, S. M. Behavioral treatment of obesity: a two-year follow-up. *Behav. Res. Ther.*, **11**, 647 B, C, D
43. Harris, M. B and Hallbauer, E. S. Self-directed weight control through eating and exercise. *Behav. Res. Ther.*, **11**, 523 B, D
44. Jordan, H. A. and Levitz, L. S. Behavior modification in a self-help group. *J. Amer. Diet. Assn.*, **62**, 27 C, D
45. Mahoney, M. J. Self-reward and self-monitoring techniques for weight control. *Behav. Ther.*, **5**, 48 B, C, D
46. Mahoney, M., Maura, N. B. and Wade, T. C. The relative efficacy of self-reward, self-punishment and self-monitoring techniques for weight loss. *J. Consult. Clin. Psychol*, **40**, 404 B, C, D
47. Martin, J. E. and Sachs, D. A. The effects of a self-control weight loss program on an obese woman. *J. Behav. Ther. Exper. Psychiat.*, **4**, 155 D
48. Romanczyk, R. G., Tracey, D. A., Wilson, G. T. and Thorpe, G. L. Behavioral techniques in the treatment of obesity: a

comparative analysis. *Behav. Res. Ther.*, **11**, 629 A, B, C, D

49. Wijesinghe, B. Massed electrical aversion treatment of compulsive eating. *J. Behav. Ther. Exper. Psychiat.*, **4**, 133 A

1974 and In Press

50. Levitz, L. S. and Stunkard, A. J. A coalition for the treatment of obesity: behavior modification and patient self-help. *Amer. J. Psychiat*, **131**, 423 C, D
51. Hagen, R. L. Group therapy versus bibliotherapy in weight reduction. *Behav. Ther.*, **5**, 222 C, D
52. Abrams, J. L. and Allen, G. H. Comparative effectiveness of situational programming, financial reinforcers and group pressure in weight reduction. *Behav. Ther.* (In Press) B, C, D
53. Bellack, A. S., Rozensky, R. and Schwartz, J. A comparison of two forms of self-monitoring in a behavioural weight reduction program. *Behav. Ther.* (In Press) D

Appendix 2

Instructions to Patients for Record Keeping

DAILY FOOD INTAKE RECORD

The accompanying list furnishes specific instructions about the daily food intake record. The food intake records are essential and it is very important that they are filled out as accurately and completely as possible. Do not leave any column blank.

Please be sure to record the starting and stopping times as exactly as possible (i.e., 9:02—9:27; not 9:00—9:30).

Fill out the records just prior to or just after eating. Carry the daily record with you. If for some reason you forget your record, jot down the information on a slip of paper or even a paper napkin and transfer the information to the food record when possible. Memory is not perfect, and if you are to become fully aware of the details of your eating it is essential that the food records be filled out at the time of eating.

A completed daily food record is provided as a sample.

At this time, your only objective is to accurately record the conditions associated with your eating. Such information provides the basis for treatment. Thus, it is critically important that the information be as accurate as possible.

It is very unwise to record only those ingestions you consider to be "good" (however you define it). We must learn about the conditions under which overeating occurs if you are to be helped by this form of treatment.

Appendix 2 was written by Henry A. Jordan, M.D., Leonard S. Lovitz, Ph.D. and Gordon M. Kimbrell, Ph.D.

Therefore, be sure you write down the information asked for every time you eat.

INSTRUCTIONS FOR COMPLETING FOOD RECORD

1. *Time:* Record the time you begin and the time you finish each meal or snack in the appropriate time block on the record form. Record the time as exactly as possible; e.g., 8:02—8:14, not 8:00—8:15. An entry should be considered a separate meal or snack if there has been a lapse of 15 minutes between bites.
2. *Place:* Record the place where you are eating. If at home—the specific room; if away from home—the place (restaurant, car, store, office, friends home, etc.) and whether at a counter, table, desk, etc.
3. *Physical position:* Use the following code: Standing (1), Sitting (2), Lying Down (3).
4. *With whom:* If alone write alone. If with one or more people, the number and relationship, i.e., husband, child, friend, strangers, etc.
5. *Associated activity:* Record anything that you're doing while eating such as reading, watching TV, talking, cooking, etc. If not engaged in any other activity, write in "eating only."
6. *Mood:* Record your mood before you begin eating. Use the first letter of whichever word most clearly coincides with your mood from the following list: Neutral, Content, Tense, Depressed, Angry, Happy, Bored, Fatigued, Rushed.
7. *Hunger:* Record your subjective feeling of hunger just *before eating.* Write down any number between 0 and 5 which describes your degree of hunger. 0 represents no hunger and 5 represents extreme hunger.
8. *Food and amount:* Record the name of the food and an estimate of either the weight of the food, the size of the portion or the number of pieces, so that caloric values may be determined.
9. *Meals:* Place an (M) next to those entries which you consider meals.
10. *Calories:* Look up the number of calories in the foods you eat. We recommend the use of two pocket-size calorie books—one which lists brand name foods and another which lists fresh foods. Use the same books through the week. Record calories for every meal and snack.
11. At the bottom of each sheet, circle the number which corresponds most accurately with the percentage of entries made at the immediate time of ingestion (including just prior to or just after).

Date: ____________ FOOD INTAKE RECORD Name: ____________

Time Start End	Place	Phys. pos.	Alone or with whom	Assoc. activity	M	H	Food and amount	Calories
6—11								
11-4								
4-9								
9-6								

Percent of entries filled out right before or after eating 0 25 50 75 100

FILLING OUT THE ANALYSIS FORM

The analysis form is very important throughout the treatment program because it provides a summary or overview of your week's eating patterns. The analysis form serves three purposes:

(1) Initially, it provides essential information for planning individualized treatment techniques

(4) As treatment continues, it is helpful in assessing the effectiveness of these treatment techniques for you.

(5) Finally, it can help you learn how to analyze your own eating habits and the factors responsible for them.

Your daily food records provide the information you need to fill out the weekly analysis form. Filling out the analysis form is not difficult, but it does require a certain amount of attention to detail. Some people like to fill out the analysis form at the end of the week, while others like to enter the data from the daily food records every day or every other day. In either case, the analysis form should include all the information from the entire week's worth of food records.

Most of the categories (I—IX) on the analysis form ask for simple frequency counts. The easiest way to record these is to use tick marks in the appropriate places to tally the total frequency. It is helpful to group the tic marks in groups of five with a diagonal being used to indicate the fifth entry (i.e. ~~////~~ // = 7).

Category I (*Time of Eating*) is a frequency count and requires that the data be entered in the form of a histogram. For each ingestion (each meal or snack), darken the square corresponding to the time interval during

I. Time of Eating

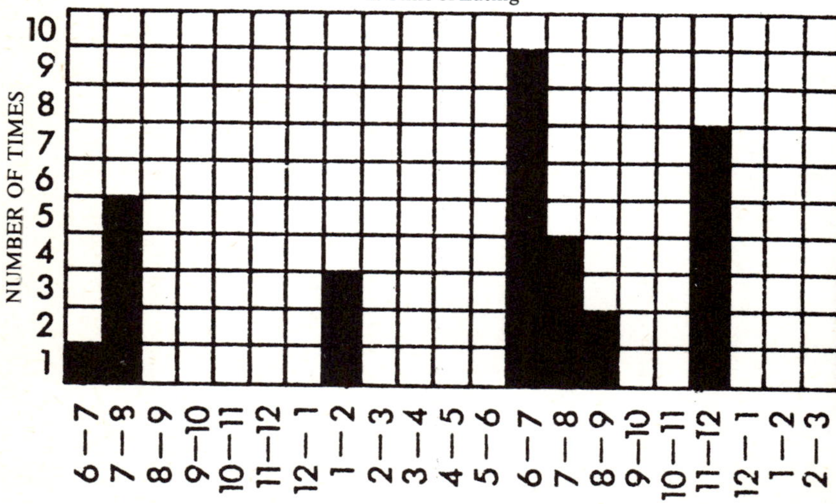

which the meal or snack started. The time intervals are plotted along the bottom of the graph (starting at 6:00 a.m.). "Number of Times" refers to the number of times during the week that a meal or snack occurred at each particular time interval.

Category I does not distinguish between meals and snacks. In this example we can see that one ingestion began sometime during the hour of 6—7 a.m., 5 between 7—8 a.m., 3 between 1—2 p.m., 9 between 6—7 p.m.,4 between 7—8 p.m., 2 between 8—9 p.m., and 7 between 11—12 midnight.

Category I provides a pictorial description of the temporal characteristics of eating for the entire week.

This is very helpful in that it provides a quick overview of both the frequency and temporal pattern of all your ingestions for the week.

For the rest of the categories (II—IX), it is necessary to analyze meals and snacks separately. This is easily done as can be seen in the example from category II.

Category II (*Duration of Eating*) asks for a count of the number of meals which lasted from 0—4 minutes, 5—10 minutes, etc. The same information is required for snacks.

II. *Duration of Eating*	*Meals*	*Snacks*
0—4 minutes	/ / /	~~////~~ ~~////~~ / /
5—10 minutes	~~////~~ / / /	~~////~~ /
11—20 minutes	/ /	/ /
Over 20 minutes	/ / /	/

Thus we can easily see that during the week, this person had 3 meals which lasted from 0—4 minutes, 8 which lasted from 5—10 minutes, 2 which lasted from 11—20 minutes and 3 which lasted over 2 minutes. There were also 12 snacks lasting 0—4 minutes, 6 snacks lasting 5—10 minutes, 2 snacks lasting from 11—20 minutes and one which lasted over 20 minutes.

Category III (*Place of Eating*) concerns the places in which meals or snacks occur. Again, it is sufficent to use tic marks to tally the frequencies.

III. *Place of Eating*	*MEALS*	*SNACKS*
Kitchen	~~////~~ / /	~~////~~
Dining Room	/ /	
Living Room		
Bedroom		
Den		/ / /

Car	/	
Bus, Train		
Walking		/
Office	/	/ / /
Restaurant	/ / / /	
Friend's home	/	
Other		~~////~~ ~~////~~ / / /

In this example, it can be seen that during the week the individual had 7 meals in the kitchen, 2 in the dining room, 1 in the car, 1 in the office, 4 in restaurants, and 1 at a friend's home. Five snacks were eaten in the kitchen, 3 in the den, 1 while walking, 3 at the office, and 13 are listed as other. Other is meant to include all places of eating not covered by the listings. Since this individual's "other" was a regular place of eating (his basement workshop) rather than a number of miscellaneous places, it is worth noting by writing it in on the analysis form.

Category IV (*Physical Position*) is a frequency count of the physical position entries on the daily food records.

IV. *Phsyical Position*	*MEALS*	*SNACKS*
(1) Standing		~~////~~ / /
(2) Sitting	~~////~~ ~~////~~ / / /	/
(3) Lying Down	/	~~////~~

In this example, it can be seen that during the week the individual ate 13 meals seated and one while lying down. Seven snacks were eaten while standing, 1 while seated and 5 while lying down.

Category V (*Alone or with Whom*) asks for a frequency count of the number of meals eaten alone, with spouse, etc. Likewise the same information is needed for snacks.

V. *Alone or with Whom*	*MEALS*	*SNACKS*
Alone	/ /	~~////~~ ~~////~~ / /
Spouse	/ /	~~////~~
Family	~~////~~ / /	/ /
Friends	/	~~////~~ /
Business Associates	/ /	/
Strangers	/ / / /	
Other		/

Each meal or snack should be counted only once. For example, a meal with your spouse and children would be entered as "family" as shown above.

In this example, it can be seen that during the week the individual had 2 meals alone, 2 with spouse, 8 with family, etc.

Category VI (*Associated Activity*) asks for a tally of the activities associated with meals and snacks.

VI. *Associated Activity*	*MEALS*	*SNACKS*
Eating Only	/ / /	
Talking	~~////~~ /	
Reading	/	/ / /
Radio, Music	/ / /	/ /
Television	~~////~~	~~////~~ / / /
Cooking		
Other (school work)		~~////~~ ~~////~~ ~~////~~ / /

In this example, the individual used "other" to separate school work from recreational reading. If you are doing more than one activity while eating, you may enter a tic mark for each.

Here it can be seen that the individual had 3 meals while doing nothing other than eating, 6 accompanied by talking, etc. Three snacks were had while reading, 2 while listening to music, etc.

Category VII (*Mood*) is a tally of the *dominant* mood (from the food record) associated with each meal or snack.

VII. *Mood*	*MEALS*	*SNACKS*
Neutral	/ / /	/ / /
Content	/ / /	
Happy	~~////~~	~~////~~ /
Tense	/	
Depressed		/
Angry		
Bored	/	/ / / /
Fatigued	/	~~////~~ / /
Rushed	/	

Category VIII (*Degree of Hunger*) asks for a frequency count of the degree of hunger experienced at each meal or snack during the week.

VIII *Degree of Hunger*	*MEALS*	*SNACKS*
0—2 (none to mild)	~~////~~ / / /	~~////~~ ~~////~~ / /
3—5 (mild to extreme	~~////~~ / /	~~////~~ / / /

Category IX (*Type of Food*) asks for a count of the number of meals or snacks during the week which involved the listed foods. The food list is partially reproduced below.

IX. *Type of Food*	*MEALS*	*SNACKS*
Alcohol	/ / /	~~////~~ / / /
Baked Goods		
Cake, Cookies, Crackers, etc.	~~////~~ ~~////~~ / /	
Candy	/	~~////~~ / /
Cheese	/ /	/ / /
Ice Cream, Sherbert	/ /	/
Jam	/ / /	
Jello	/	/
Nuts		~~////~~ / / /
Peanut Butter	/	/ /
Potato Chips, etc.	/	/ / / /
Pretzels		/
Sodas		
Diet	/ /	/ / / /
Regular	/	/ / /
Sugar	/ /	
Coffee-mate	~~////~~	~~////~~ ~~////~~ /

It is important to point out that the amount of each food does not enter into this. Thus, in the above example, it can be seen that 7 snacks involved candy. This does not take into account the number of pieces of candy eaten during each of these seven snacks. It does not mean that 7 pieces of candy were eaten.

Category IX provides a quick overview of food selection for the week. If it is necessary to determine the amount consumed of selected food, it is easily done by reviewing the daily food records.

For Category X (*Total caloric intake*) add up the total calories consumed each day and enter the total in the appropriate place.

X. *Total Caloric Intake*

Friday *1500* Saturday *2125* Sunday *4100* Monday *875*
Tuesday *1250* Wednesday *1460* Thursday *1800*

Category XI (*Techniques*) is for you to record the special techniques which you have been asked to try during the week. This will not be used during the first 3 or 4 weeks of the program.

XI. *Techniques*

(1) ______________________________

(2) ______________________________

(3) ______________________________

(4) ______________________________

GENERAL CONSIDERATIONS

From the above comments and examples, you can see that it is very important to fill out your daily food records completely and accurately. The weekly analysis form is easy and straight forward.

It is generally easier to transfer all the data concerning each ingestion to the analysis form rather than go through all your records entering data on time of eating; then going back and entering data on duration, etc. One tends to lose one's place all too easily. Many people find it helpful to make a check mark in the margin after entering all the data for a given ingestion. in case the telephone rings or they are distracted for some reason.

The following example shows how this might be done for one sample ingestion.

EXAMPLE

Time Start	Time End	Place	Phys. Pos.	Alone or with whom	Assoc. Activity	M	H	Food and Amount	Calories
6-11									
7:43	7:51	kitchen	2	alone	reading	H	S	2 cups corn flakes 1 cup milk, whole (M) 2 slices toast 1 TBS butter	✓ 190 175 130 100

In the above example, one square in the 7—8 a.m. time interval would be darkened. One tic mark would be placed under each of the following categories II (5—10 minutes), III. (kitchen), IV. (sitting), V. (alone), VI.

BEHAVIORAL WEIGHT CONTROL PROGRAM

ANALYSIS OF FOOD INTAKE

I. Time of Eating

NUMBER OF TIMES	6—7	7—8	8—9	9—10	10—11	11—12	12—1	1—2	2—3	3—4	4—5	5—6	6—7	7—8	8—9	9—10	10—11	11—12	12—1	1—2	2—3
10																					
9																					
8																					
7																					
6																					
5																					
4																					
3																					
2																					
1																					

II. Duration of Eating

	MEALS	SNACKS
0-4 Minutes		
5-10 Minutes		
11-20 Minutes		
Over 20 Minutes		

III. Place of Eating

Kitchen		
Dining Room		
Living Room		
Bedroom		
Den		
Car		
Bus, Train		
Walking		

Place of Eating (Cont.)

Office		
Restaurant		
Friend's Home		
Other		

IV. Physical Position

Standing		
Sitting		
Lying Down		

V. Alone or With Whom

Alone		
Spouse		
Family		
Friends		
Business Associates		
Strangers		
Other		

VI. Associated Activity

Eating Only		
Talking		
Reading		
Radio, Music		
Television		
Cooking		
Other		

VII. Mood

Neutral		
Content		
Happy		
Tense		
Depressed		
Angry		
Bored		
Fatigued		
Rushed		

VIII. Degree of Hunger

0-2 (None to Mild)		
3-5 (Mild to Extreme)		

IX. Type of Food

Alcohol		
Baked Goods		
Cake, Cookies, Crackers, etc.		
Candy		
Cheese		
Ice Cream, Sherbert		
Jam		
Jello		
Nuts		
Peanut Butter		
Potato Chips, etc.		
Pretzels		
Sodas		
Diet		
Regular		
Sugar		
Coffee-mate		

Type of Food (Cont.)

Bread, Rolls		
Butter, Margerine		
Margarine		
Cereal		
Condiments		
Eggs		
Fish		
Fruit		
Juice		
Mayonnaise		
Meat		
Milk		
Whole		
Skim		
Pasta Products		
Pizza		
Potatoes		
Poultry		
Salads		
Salad Dressing		
Soup		
Syrups, Sauces		
Vegetables		
Waffles, Pancakes		
Yogurt, Cottage Ch.		

X. Total Caloric Intake

Friday ________ Saturday ________ Sunday ____

Mon. ________ Tues. ________ Wed. ________ Thurs. ____

XI. Techniques

1. ____________________
2. ____________________
3. ____________________
4. ____________________

Date:____________ DAILY ACTIVITY RECORD Name:____________

	:00 :15 a b c	:15 :30 a b c	:30 :45 a b c	:45 :60 a b c		:00 :15 a b c	:15 :30 a b c	:30 :45 a b c	:45 :60 a b c
6 A.M.					6 P.M.				
7 A.M.					7 P.M.				
8 A.M.					8 P.M.				
9 A.M.					9 P.M.				
10 A.M.					10 P.M.				
11 A.M.					11 P.M.				
12 A.M.					12 P.M.				
					1 A.M.				
2 P.M.					2 A.M.				
3 P.M.					3 A.M.				
4 P.M.					4 A.M.				
5 P.M.					5 A.M.				

ANALYSIS TABLE

	0	1	2	3	4
a					
b					
c					

(reading), VII. (Happy), VIII. (Hunger 3—5), IX (cereal, milk-whole, bread and butter). All entries in categories II—IX go in the MEALS column since the food record indicates that this ingestion is to be regarded as a meal. The check mark in the "calories" column means that all the data has been entered on the analysis form.

Finally, be sure to put your name and the date of the session at which the information is in the upper right hand corner of the analysis form. Make sure that your name and each day's date is on the daily food record sheets.

REFERENCES

1. Stunkard, A. J. and McLaren-Hume, M. (1959). The results of treatment for obesity. A review of the literature and report of a series. *Arch. Intern. Med.,* **103,** 79
2. Sohar, E. and Sneh, E. (1973). Follow-up of obese patients: 14 years after a successful reducing diet. *Amer. J. Clin. Nutr.,* **26,** 845
3. Keys, A., Brozek, J., Henschel, A., Mickelsen, O. and Taylor, H. L. L. (1950). *The Biology of Human Starvation.* Vols. 1 and 2. (Minneapolis: Univ. of Minnesota Press)
4. Sims, E. A. H., Goldman, R. F., Gluck, C. M., Horton, E. S., Kelleher, P. C. and Rowe, D. W. (1968). Experimental obesity in man. *Trans. Assoc. Amer. Physicians,* **81,** 153
5. Miller, D. S. and Mumford, P. (1967). Gluttony. 1. An experimental study of overeating low- or high-protein diets. *Amer. J. Clin. Nutr.,* **20,** 1212
6. Jordan, H. A. (1973). In defense of body weight, *J. Amer. Diet Ass.,* **62,** 1, 17
7. Stunkard, A. J. (1957). The 'dieting depression': Incidence and clinical characteristics of untoward responses to weight reduction regimens. *Amer. J. Med.,* **23,** 77
8. Glucksman, M. L., Hirsh, J. (1968). The response of obese patients to weight reduction: A clinical evaluation of behavior. *Psychosom. Med.,* **30,** 1
9. Bray, G. A. (1969). Effect of caloric restriction on energy expenditure in obese patients. *Lancet,* **ii,** 397
10. Bruch, H. (1973). *Eating Disorders: Obesity, Anorexia Nervosa, and the Person Within.* (New York; Basic Books, Inc.)
11. Krasner, L. and Ullmann, L. P. (1973). *Behavior Influence and Personality.* (New York: Holt, Rinehart and Winston, Inc.)
12. Brillat-Savarin, J. a. (1971). *The Physiology of Taste.* (Transl. from French by Fisher, M. F. K.) (New York: Alfred A. Knopf)

13. Hirsch, J. and Knittle, J. L. (1970). Cellularity of obese and nonobese human adipose tissue. *Fed. Proc.,* **29,** 1516
14. Abramson, E. E. A review of behavioral approaches to weight control. *Behav. Res. Ther.,* **11,** 547
15. Hall, S. M. and Hall, R. G. Outcome and methodological considerations in the behavioral treatment of obesity. *Behav. Ther.* (In Press).
16. Stuart, R. B. Behavioral control of overeating: a status report. In Proceedings of the Fogarty International Center Conference on Obesity, Washington, D.C. (G. A. Bray, editor) National Institute of Health (In Press)
17. Stunkard, A. J. (1972). New therapies for the eating disorders: behavior modification of obesity and anorexia nervosa. *Arch. Gen. Psychiat.,* **26,** 391
18. Young, C. M., Moore, N. S., Berresford, K., Einset, B. M. and Waldner, B. G. (1955). The problem of the obese patient. *J. Amer. Diet Ass,* **31,** 1111
19. Kanfer, F. H. (1970). Self regulation: Research issues and speculations. *In Behavior Modification in Clinical psychology.* (Neuringer, C. and Michael, J. L., editors) (New York: Appleton-Century-Crofts)
20. Mahoney, M. (1972). Research issues in self-management. *Behav. Ther.,* **3,** 45
21. Bellack, A. S., Rozensky, R and Schwartz, J. A comparison of two forms of self-monitoring in a behavioral weight reduction program. *Behav. Ther.* (In Press)

7

Anorectic Drugs

Trevor Silverstone

INTRODUCTION

Anorectic drugs, as their name implies, are substances which, when given in adequate dosage, produce a state of anorexia, a condition defined as 'being without appetite'; indeed, anorectic drugs are often called 'appetite suppressants'. The term 'appetite' refers to an individual's tendency to experience 'hunger', a state which, in turn, may be defined as 'the desire to eat'; hunger being generally regarded as a more immediate sensation than appetite. Hunger can change from hour to hour whereas appetite, although also referring to the desire for food, is usually used in a context where change is less rapid.

As with many significant advances in clinical pharmacology, the first indication that a centrally acting drug might affect hunger, and thus help obese patients lose weight arose largely by chance. Amphetamine, a phenylethylamine compound, had originally been synthesised by Alles in 1927 to provide a cheaper, synthetic substitute for ephedrine[1]. It was soon found to be a potent central stimulant. This property was applied clinically in the treatment of narcolepsy[2] and some of those treated were noted to lose weight[3,4]. Davidoff and Reifenstein[5] consequently suggested that amphetamine '. . . may be of use in reducing weight'. This suggestion was soon taken up enthusiastically by Lesses and Myerson[6] who were extremely gratified by the response they obtained in obese patients: '. . . on the one hand it decreases the appetite, and on the other so increases the sense of well being and of energy that physical activity is spontaneously increased'.

So began what has become an ever increasing interest on the part of clinicians, pharmacologists and physiologists in the quest for appetite reducing drugs to help obese patients to eat less, and thus lose weight. By 1941, that is a mere six years after the first clinical application of amphetamine, there were already over 300 published papers and reviews referring to it[7]. Since then a number of other centrally acting phenylethylamine compounds have been introduced as appetite

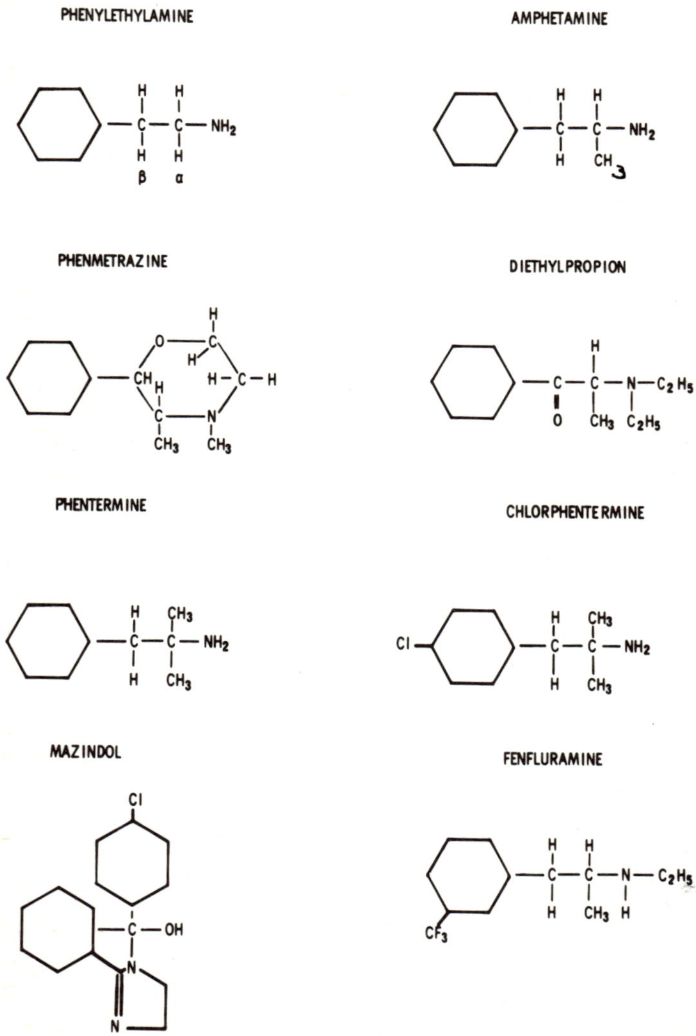

FIGURE 7.1 Formulae of anorectic drugs

suppressants. These include: phenmetrazine (Preludin); phentermine (Duromine); diethylpropion (Tenuate, Tepanil, Apisate); chlorphentermine (Lucofen, Presate); and fenfluramine (Ponderax, Ponderal, Pondomin) (Figure 7.1). In addition there are a number of non-phenylethylamine compounds which are claimed to have anorectic properties: (*a*) mazindol (Teronac, Sanorex); (*b*) the biguanide compounds (metformin (glucophage) and phenformin (Dibotin)); (*c*) glucagon, (*d*) chorionic gonadotrophin and (*e*) bulk agents such as methyl cellulose and guar gum which are presumed to produce satiety by swelling in the stomach.

Before going on to discuss the clinical applications of these drugs and deciding which, if any, have a place in the treatment of obesity, I think it would be useful to spend some time considering whether the drugs listed do, in fact, reduce appetite.

ANORECTIC ACTIVITY

Strictly speaking one can only speak of hunger and appetite in relation to man. Observations on the eating behaviour of experimental animals are necessarily limited to descriptions of the eating itself, and no firm conclusions may be drawn from such observations about these animals' subjective state. Only human subjects can say whether or not they feel more or less hungry under different conditions. Therefore we can only really tell whether a given drug has an effect on appetite by testing it in man.

Hunger, in common with other subjective variables, cannot be measured directly, although it can be quantified. Using a linear analogue scale (Figure 7.2) a valid assessment can be made of the degree

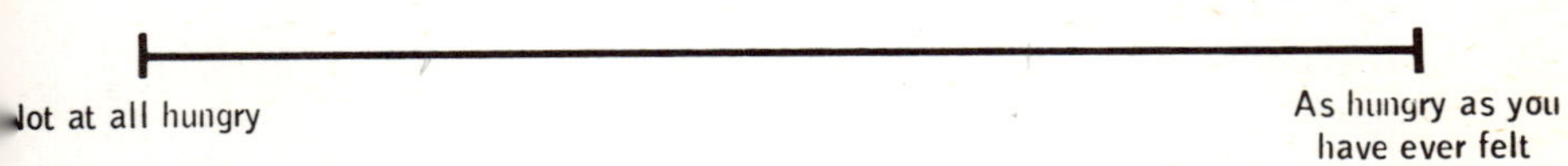

FIGURE 7.2 Linear visual analogue hunger rating scale

of hunger experienced by a given individual at a particular time as compared with that same person's hunger at another time[8]. The subject is instructed to mark the scale at the point which seems appropriate to him at the given time; on a subsequent occasion he is asked to mark a similar scale in the same way. It is assumed that if he feels hungrier on the second occasion than on the first, the second scale would be marked more towards the right than the first, and *vice versa*. Defining hunger as 'the desire to eat' and comparing the hunger rating of the same individual at a number of meals with the amount he actually eats, a significant correlation between hunger and food intake can be obtained (Figure 7.3). This confirms the belief that hunger ratings do reflect the desire to eat within an individual.

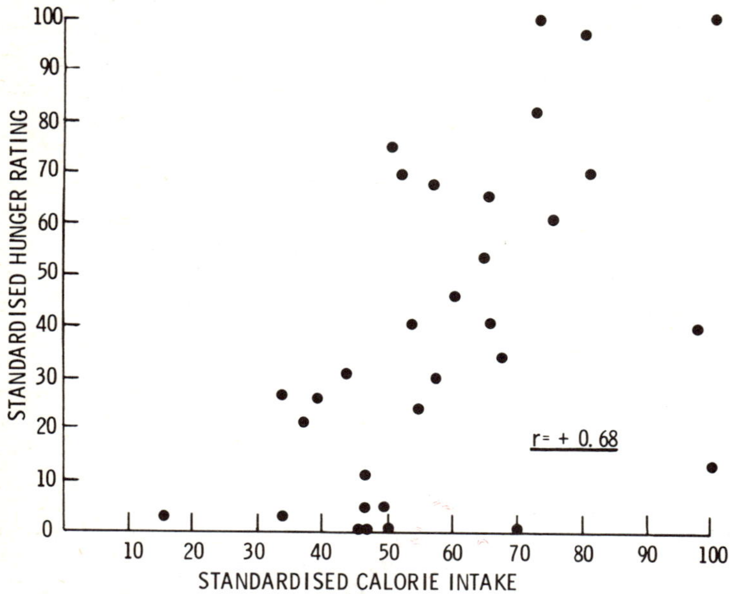

FIGURE 7.3 Correlation between standardised hunger ratings (each individual's score is expressed as a percentage of his maximum score) and standardised food intake (expressed in the same way as hunger rating)

A. Phenylethylamine derivatives

1. D-amphetamine sulphate

Although several reports indicated that racemic amphetamine and d-amphetamine sulphate reduced hunger, it was not clear to what degree this occurred in clinical practice. On the one hand were the glowing accounts of Lesses and Myerson[6] and others indicating that amphetamine almost invariably produced such a profound anorexia that keeping to a reducing diet was child's play; on the other hand there were indications that it was only relatively few patients who experienced any significant anorexia, and amphetamine was of little help in keeping to a diet[9].

Among normal weight subjects, as among the obese, the anorectic response to amphetamine and d-amphetamine is variable. In an early controlled investigation of Danish office workers Bahnsen *et al.*[10] found that a single dose of amphetamine (20 mg for men and 10 mg for women) produced an anorectic effect in only 20%, although this was much greater than the 1% who noted a similar effect with placebo. A similar variability of anorectic response among normal subjects was reported by Jacobson and Woolstein[11]. Harris *et al.*[12] showed that amphetamine caused both obese and normal subjects to eat less, but they did not evaluate hunger directly; nevertheless they confidently attributed the weight loss they observed to anorexia.

Bernstein and Grossman[13] could find no consistent effect on hunger within thirty minutes of 10 mg amphetamine administered through a gastric tube. In contrast, using the linear analogue scale already described, Stunkard and I found that 10 mg d-amphetamine, when compared with placebo, did produce a statistically significant fall in

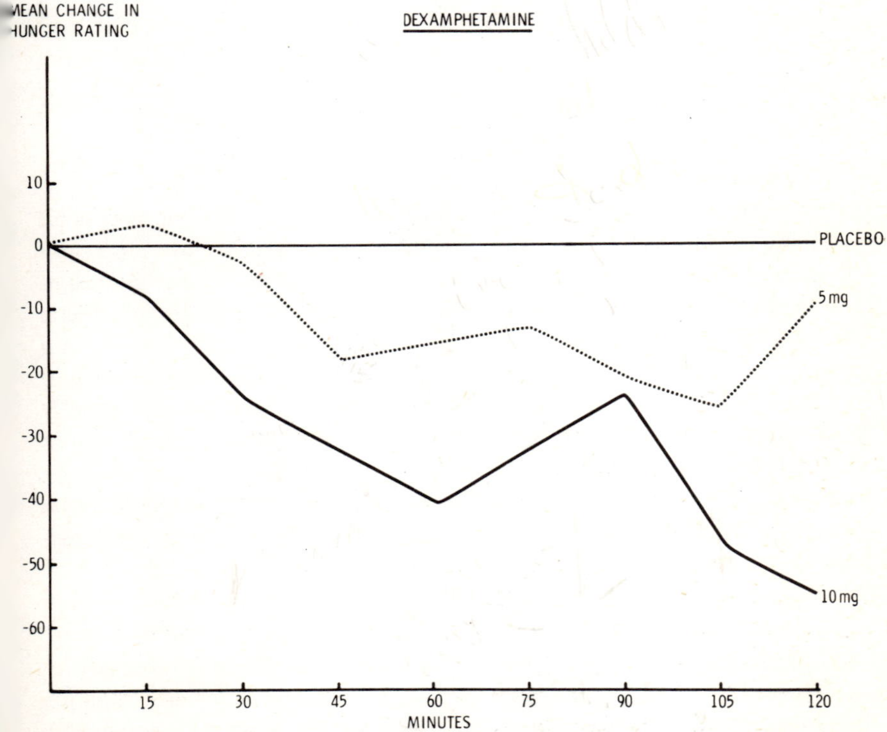

FIGURE 7.4 The mean effect of a single oral dose of 5 mg and 10 mg d-amphetamine on the change in hunger ratings in eight fasting normal male subjects over a two hour period compared with changes in hunger ratings occurring in a similar period after placebo administration

subjective hunger ratings; the maximal effect occurring two hours after administration (Figure 7.4). There was a corresponding reduction in calorie intake[14]; 5 mg was less effective. It would appear, therefore, that d-amphetamine sulphate does have a true anorectic effect which is maximal some two to three hours after administration.

2. Phenmetrazine

Clinical studies with phenmetrazine suggested that it too had a direct anorectic effect[15]. However, using a crude 'hungry'/'not hungry' rating, Penick and Hinkle[16] could detect little consistent anorectic effect of phenmetrazine 25 mg in normal subjects. This was perhaps too blunt a rating to detect the effect of relatively small doses, and clinical observations suggest that it is likely that the anorectic potential of phenmetrazine is similar to that of amphetamine[17].

3. Phentermine

As with the drugs already considered, the claimed anorectic potential of phentermine was originally based on clinical impressions[18,19]. A more critical evaluation of the anorectic action of phentermine using the linear analogue scale has confirmed these clinical impressions[20].

4. Diethylpropion

Early clinical reports[21,22] indicated that the effect of diethylpropion on reducing food intake and thereby producing weight loss in obese patients was probably based on an anorectic effect. Using a design similar to that employed in the quantitative evaluation of the anorectic activity of d-amphetamine, I found that a single dose of 50 mg diethylpropion, but not 25 mg, reduced hunger significantly in normal male subjects[23] (Figure 7.5). In addition, assessment, under strictly controlled conditions, of the anorectic activity of the long-acting form of diethylpropion (Tenuate Dospan) in eighteen moderately overweight young women, again using the linear analogue scale, revealed that the drug significantly reduced hunger ratings and correspondingly reduced food intake[24].

5. Chlorphentermine

Although the presumption has been made that chlorphentermine acts as an anorectic in producing weight loss in obese patients[25,26], this has not been evaluated directly. Therefore the relative anorectic potency of chlorphentermine in man is undetermined at present. Animal data[27] would suggest that it was approximately equivalent to diethylpropion in reducing food intake.

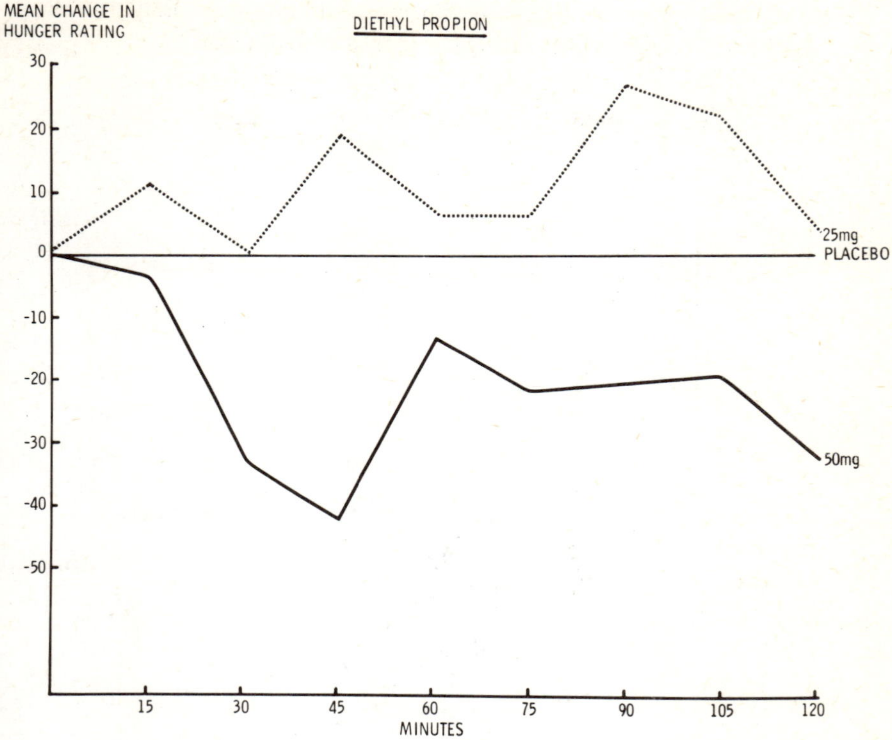

FIGURE 7.5 The mean effect of a single oral dose of 25 mg and 50 mg diethylpropion on the change in hunger ratings in eight fasting normal male subjects over a two hour period compared with the change in hunger ratings occurring in a similar period after placebo administration

6. *Fenfluramine*

The efficacy of fenfluramine, the most recently introduced of the phenylethylamine anorectic drugs in the treatment of obesity[28,29] was presumed to be due to a central appetite suppressant action; a presumption supported by other clinical studies in which appetite was enquired about routinely[30].

In an acute study in normal subjects using a linear analogue scale fenfluramine was found to reduce hunger significantly[31]. Of the doses studied the 80 mg dose produced the greatest effect (Figure 7.6); this was accompanied by the highest blood level. From the data obtained from this and previous studies[32], it would appear that for significant anorexia to occur a plasma level of approximately 100 ng/ml is required. In a rather more prolonged study in normal subjects in which linear analogue scales were completed weekly, fenfluramine 40 mg twice daily produced a significant fall in hunger rating compared with placebo[33].

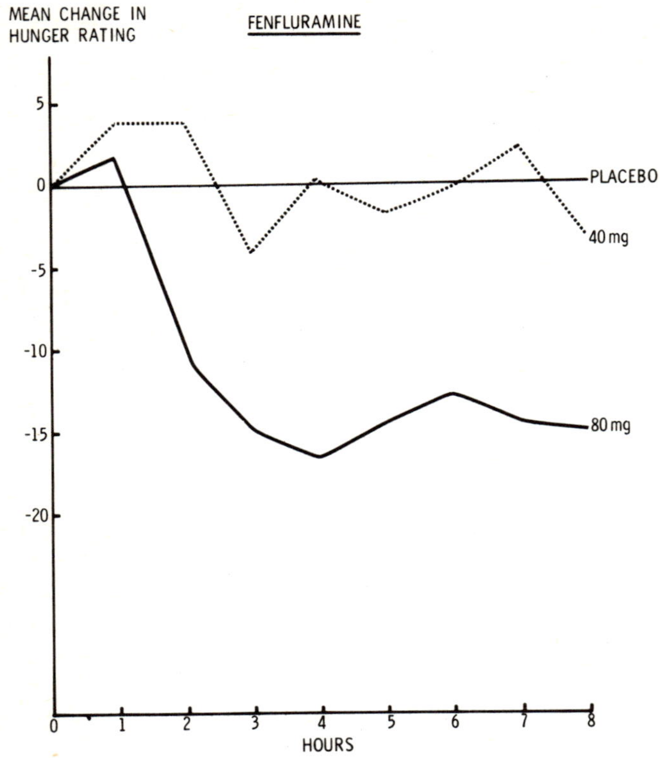

FIGURE 7.6 The mean effect of a single oral dose of 40 mg and 80 mg fenfluramine on the change in hunger ratings in eight fasting normal male subjects and eight fasting normal female subjects over an eight hour period compared with the change in hunger ratings occurring over a similar period after placebo administration

B. Other centrally-acting compounds

1. Mazindol

This recently introduced isoindole derivative which causes monkeys and other experimental animals to eat less, also produces a lowered calorie intake in obese patients. This reduction in calorie intake is attributed to a central anorectic effect of the drug and there is a certain amount of evidence from controlled clinical trials to suggest that this is so[34,35], although the magnitude of the anorectic action would appear to be somewhat variable[36]. No direct quantitative evaluation of its anorectic activity in normal subjects has yet been undertaken.

2. Chorionic gonadotrophin

Chorionic gonadotrophin was introduced for the treatment of obesity some twenty years ago by Simeons[37]. Simeons remarked on the loss of appetite it produced, an anorexia which allowed obese patients receiving daily injections of 120 i.u. to tolerate a 500 calorie diet with equanimity. Subsequent double-blind trials failed to show any superiority of injections of chorionic gonadotrophin over saline injections[38,39], and in some cases appetite was reported to have increased rather than decreased. More recently, however, an equally careful double-blind study[40] has revealed a distinct advantage for chorionic gonadotrophin in terms of anorexia, weight loss and a sense of well-being. This finding in turn has itself been questioned[41]. Whatever the relative anorectic potency of chorionic gonadotrophin its mode of action remains obscure.

C. Drugs affecting carbohydrate metabolism

1. Diguanide compounds

While the diguanide compounds metformin and phenformin alter carbohydrate metabolism in obese diabetic patients, and appear to help such patients lose weight, their value in non-diabetic obesity is less clear. Current opinion would indicate that these drugs do not have a primary anorectic effect and they are consequently relatively ineffective in the treatment of uncomplicated obesity[42,43]. In any case, metformin was found to be clearly less effective than fenfluramine in promoting weight loss; the likely inference being that it is equally less effective in reducing hunger. Even where a significant weight loss has been produced by diguanides this was not thought to be attributable to a primary anorectic action[44].

2. Glucagon

There have been very few studies of the effect of glucagon on hunger, and even fewer on its potential use as a therapeutic agent in obesity. In one experiment on four healthy male volunteers glucagon 1 mg by intramuscular injection caused previously hungry subjects to rate themselves as 'not hungry' two hours later[45]. The anorectic effect was greater than that following oral phenmetrazine 25 mg, although in the case of phenmetrazine the rating was made only an hour after ingestion; this may have been too soon to obtain a significant effect. The anorectic action of glucagon could be related to its inhibitory effect on the motor activity of the fasting stomach, or it could be centrally mediated[46].

D. Bulk agents

The idea of filling up the stomach with an inert, non-digestable bulk agent has a refreshing simplicity about it. Unfortunately trials of methyl cellulose have failed to indicate that it helps obese patients lose weight by causing them to eat less[47,48]. More direct examination of the anorectic potency of methyl cellulose in doses up to 3.375 g (nine tablets) using the linear analogue hunger scale did not reveal any hunger reducing activity whatsoever[23]. Guar gum in a similar dose was equally ineffective.

Conclusion

Thus far we may state with some confidence that at least four of the centrally acting phenylethylamines, d-amphetamine, phentermine, diethylpropion and fenfluramine have a true anorectic activity. While this activity is not very marked following a single dose, it may become more pronounced with longer periods of administration in which higher blood levels are built up. Chorionic gonadotrophin remains an enigma and will require further detailed evaluation of its potential anorectic potency, as will mazindol. The diguanides appear to have little direct anorectic action, but glucagon does. It is unknown whether this action of glucagon is secondary to a direct effect on the gastro-intestinal tract, or whether it is due to an alteration of carbohydrate metabolism, or even to a direct action on the brain.

Finally the bulk agents methyl cellulose and guar gum seem to have no effect at all on subjective hunger and are unlikely to be of any real benefit in the treatment of obesity.

POSSIBLE MECHANISMS OF ACTION

Having determined that certain of the phenylethylamines have a true anorectic action we can review the possible physiological and anatomical bases for this. Of necessity such mechanisms can only be examined in experimental animals, and in order to draw any useful conclusions from animal studies, we have to assume a relationship between anorectic activity in man and reduction in feeding in animals. That is to say, if a drug causes anorexia in man, and also produces reduction in food intake in animals, we might assume a similar mechanism to underly both events. While this assumption may seem reasonable, we can never be certain of its validity, and any conclusions we might draw from it must remain tentative.

The two drugs about which most is known in terms of pharmacology are amphetamine and fenfluramine, and these will be dealt with in some detail. Where appropriate the other phenylethylamines and mazindol will also be considered.

Before going on to discuss individual compounds it might be helpful to consider the mid-brain and diencephalic structures and systems within the brain which are thought to underly the regulation of food intake. Almost all the studies on these topics have been performed on rats; however, where such studies have been replicated in other species the findings have usually been similar.

A. Neurochemical basis of food intake

Until very recently the hypothalamus was considered to be the dominant regulating system for food intake, this area of the brain having first been implicated by the clinical findings of Mohr in 1840 and Frohlich in 1910. In the 1940s experimental observations supported the view that hypothalamic damage (particularly in the medial hypothalamus) could produce obesity[49]. In contrast, bilateral lesions in the lateral hypothalamus produced aphagia. The theory was therefore put forward that the activities of the medial and lateral hypothalamus were complementary; the medial part being referred to as the 'satiety' centre, the lateral part being called the 'feeding' centre. Stimulation studies corroborated these views, stimulation of the lateral hypothalamus causing feeding and that of the medial hypothalamus caused eating to stop. On the basis of further evidence it was suggested that the 'satiety' centre acted by suppressing the activity of the 'feeding' centre[50]. Although these hypothalamic centres were considered to be essential in the regulation of food intake it was recognised that they came under the influence of visceral nuclei in the lower brain stem as well as that of higher centres in the limbic system and the neocortex.

The supremacy of the lateral hypothalamus in regulating food intake was subsequently questioned[51,52], the alternative suggestion being made that fibres from the globus pallidus passing into the median forebrain bundle via the lateral hypothalamus were the critical pathway. More recently a further reappraisal has been made of the pathways underlying feeding[53]. A tract passing from the substantia nigra to the corpus striatum near the median forebrain bundle, which has dopamine as its mediating neurotransmitter has been found to play a major role in the regulation of feeding. In addition a more medially placed dopaminergic tract passing to the limbic system may also play an important part (Figure 7.7).

Similarly, the primacy of the ventromedial nucleus in regulating satiety has been undermined by the finding that it is the ventral noradrenergic bundle which is important, rather than the ventromedial nucleus itself[54]. Thus the concept of two discrete hypothalamic 'centres' has given way to one involving at least two pathways; one which is dopaminergic running in or near the medial forebrain bundle within the

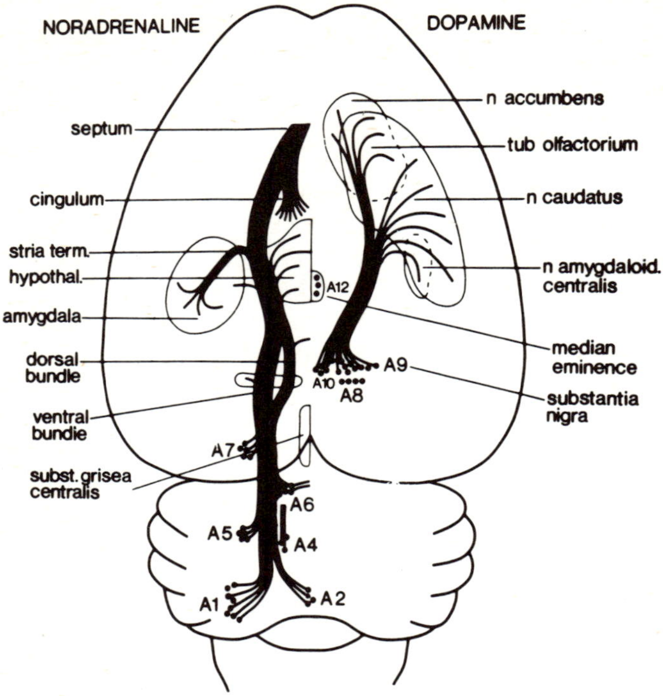

FIGURE 7.7 Dopaminergic and noradrenergic pathways in the rat brain thought to be involved in feeding behaviour (reprinted, with permission, from Ungerstedt, 1971)

lateral hypothalamus, and another which is noradrenergic, passing to the medial hypothalamus, and also at least in part running in the medial forebrain bundle[55] (Figure 7.7). In addition there are centrofugal fibres from the globus pallidus, and fibres passing from the amygdala and other limbic structures to the diencephalon which are also thought to play a part in the regulation of food intake[56,57]. The way these various areas of the brain interact to regulate feeding and the physiological signals to which they respond are, as yet, uncertain[58,59].

Central to any understanding of the way drugs act within the nervous system is a knowledge of the role played by physiological neurotransmitters. Those thought to be important in food intake regulation are noradrenaline (NA), dopamine (DA), 5-hydroxytryptamine (5HT) and perhaps acetyl choline.

There appears to be general agreement that local application of noradrenaline in the hypothalamic area causes feeding[60,61]. How this fits in with the dopaminergic feeding system is not clear. Specific DA blockers such as pimozide have no effect on eating in animals, whereas chlorpromazine, which is both an NA and DA blocker, increases feeding. This, too, is difficult to reconcile with a purely NA-induced feeding response. To complicate matters still further, *increased* feeding results from destruction of the ventral NA system (probably equivalent to what was previously called the satiety centre—see above), and some authors even deny that intrahypothalamic NA causes feeding at all[62]. However, if NA does have a facilitatory effect on feeding it is probably via an alpha adrenergic response, as it is blocked by alpha adrenergic receptor blocking drugs such as phentolamine, and not by beta adrenergic receptor blocking drugs[63]. While this may be true for rats and sheep, it may not be so for cattle[64]. Furthermore there is contrary evidence to suggest that even in rats feeding may be a beta response and not an alpha one[65].

As far as other neurotransmitters are concerned, the picture is even less clear. 5HT would appear to be involved, especially when considered in the light of fenfluramine anorexia (see below), in addition direct application of 5HT into the hypothalamus causes decreased feeding which is blocked by beta adrenergic blocking drugs[66]. Acetyl choline has been implicated in drinking regulation, but it may also have some role in feeding[67,68].

It is obvious that the situation is complex; and the view that there is a specific neurotransmitter for each given type of behaviour is likely to be an over-simplification[67].

B. Amphetamine

Racemic amphetamine consists of equal parts of the dextrorotatory (+) isomer and the laevorotatory (—) isomer. Both clinically and experimentally it has been found that the d-isomer is a more potent anorectic than the l-isomer in a ratio of approximately 3:1[69,70]. This corresponds more closely to what would be expected if amphetamine acted on a DA pathway rather than on an NA one. In keeping with this, destruction of the DA nigrostriatal tract reduces the anorectic activity of amphetamine[71,72], as does blocking of DA receptors by pimozide[73,74]. As the DA pathway itself is involved in the control of feeding, amphetamine could act by releasing DA and also blocking its re-uptake. If this were the case the DA pathway might be viewed as an anorectic rather than a hunger pathway, as the aphagia seen on bilateral destruction of the DA system is but part of a more general reduction in motor behaviour[53]. An alternative explanatory explanation involves the concept of feedback inhibition[75]. Earlier studies had indicated that amphetamine-induced anorexia was related to NA activity[61], and this still remains a possibility.

Amphetamine certainly releases NA within the hypothalamus but how this affects the situation is not clear[76]. In addition, a case has been made for an action of amphetamine on the medial hypothalamus as well as on the lateral[77]; although lesions of the medial hypothalamus increase the affect of amphetamine[78], whereas lateral hypothalamic lesions diminish amphetamine-induced anorexia[79].

C. Phenmetrazine, phentermine, diethylpropion and chlorphentermine

Phenmetrazine is thought to act on the central nervous system in a similar way to amphetamine. It (like chlorphentermine) is ineffective in chlorpromazine-induced obesity[80,81], possibly because the effect on DA release, attributed to phenmetrazine, is blocked by chlorpromazine.

Phentermine has a similar anorectic profile and sympathomimetic properties[82], but central nervous stimulation is possibly less[83].

Diethylpropion, administered systemically, was found to alter the threshold of hypothalamic stimulation required to elicit eating in rats[84]. Although the dose required to produce this was greater than that for amphetamine the effect was similar. In rats a dose of diethylpropion with an effect on food intake equivalent to amphetamine produced less central stimulation and caused no cardiovascular changes[27]. Mice, which have become obese following gold thioglucose-induced damage to the medial hypothalamus are not responsive to the anorectic effect of diethylpropion whereas they are to dexamphetamine[85]. This indicates that diethylpropion may act mainly on the medial hypothalamic area in contrast to amphetamine which is thought to act mainly on the lateral hypothalamus (see above). Thus while there may be similarities between amphetamine and diethylpropion there are also significant differences.

In contrast to the other compounds discussed thus far, chlorphentermine causes little central nervous stimulation[86,87] and appears to be pharmacologically more similar to fenfluramine than to amphetamine[27].

D. Fenfluramine

Fenfluramine, unlike amphetamine, causes reduction in the food intake of experimental animals even after lesions in the dopaminergic feeding pathway within the hypothalamus; if anything, the anorectic effect is enhanced by such lesions[88]. In contrast lesions involving the 5HT system in the mid brain raphé markedly reduced the effect of fenfluramine on food intake in rats[89]. Furthermore 5HT receptor blocking drugs such as methysergide[90,91] and cyproheptadine also interfere with the action of fenfluramine on feeding. On the basis of this and other evidence it is thought that fenfluramine acts both by increasing 5HT release from the presynaptic neurones and by reducing 5HT re-uptake from the synapse[92]. In keeping with this viewpoint is the finding that drugs such as clomipramine which block the membrane pump in 5HT neurones also counter the effects of fenfluramine on feeding, suggesting that fenfluramine shares the same uptake mechanism as 5HT[93]. Imipramine, which reduces NA re-uptake (but not 5HT) has no such effect on fenfluramine activity. Finally, chlorpromazine-induced obesity is countered by fenfluramine[94] in contrast to other anorectic drugs, again suggesting a different mode of action.

There would therefore seem to be a 5HT-mediated mechanism involved in the regulation of food intake which is the site at which fenfluramine exerts its effect.

In addition to its central anorectic action fenfluramine may have a direct metabolic effect. This has been shown to occur in isolated human muscle[95], and in a human forearm preparation[96]. The significance of this in the treatment of human obesity is unclear as careful metabolic measurements have failed to reveal any weight loss over and above that explicable in terms of a reduced food intake[97,98]. There is also the possibility that fenfluramine reduces the absorption of triglycerides[99], but whether this has any clinical relevance is not known.

E. Mazindol

Mazindol, an isoindol derivative, is said to block the re-uptake of NA within the central nervous system[100], and in this respect is similar to the tricyclic antidepressant imipramine. How this action could produce an anorectic effect is unclear—if hypothalamic NA causes feeding (see above), increased availability of NA should stimulate rather than inhibit feeding activity. But, if the satiety pathway is NA-mediated (see above) increased availability of NA could lead to a reduction in food intake. There is also a report suggesting that mazindol facilitates electrical activity in the septal area[100]; again, the relevance of this to feeding behaviour is uncertain. Mazindol also appears to have a direct DA stimulating activity. Its anorectic action could thus be explained in the light of potentiation of the DA pathway.

CLINICAL APPLICATIONS

Before any drug can be shown to be useful clinically it should fulfill the following criteria:

(i) It must be safe—this is usually determined in the first instance on the basis of animal toxicological studies; subsequent human toxicological investigations are required to confirm that it is equally safe in man.

(ii) It should possess a pharmacological action in man which supports its use in the condition to be treated.

(iii) Evidence of its efficacy in the relevant clinical condition is required. Initial clinical screening followed by adequate double blind studies comparing the efficacy of the drug in question to that of a placebo of identical appearance is usually needed to determine this point.

(iv) The drug in question should be as effective and acceptable as other available remedies.

(v) Potential long-term disadvantages should be minimal.

In the case of the anorectic drugs thus far considered, certain of them are found wanting in one or more of these criteria, particularly in those relating to pharmacological activity (criterion ii) and to long term disadvantages (criterion v).

We have already seen how the bulk agents containing methyl cellulose or guar gum[25], and the diguanide compounds[45], fail to show any specific anorectic activity. Chorionic gonadotrophin may possess some anorectic activity but there is considerable contention about this[40,41].

Amphetamine and phenmetrazine, while possessing definite anorectic properties, produce marked central stimulation effects in man[101,102] which have led to psychological dependence developing in a number of cases of obesity treated with these drugs[103]. They have also been employed as drugs of abuse by susceptible individuals[103,104]. In some cases such abuse has led to the drugs being taken in doses large enough to produce a frank paranoid psychosis[104-109]. Because of these serious potential hazards neither amphetamine nor phenmetrazine can be recommended for the treatment of obesity[110]. In fact many physicians consider that the use of amphetamine and phenmetrazine should be severely curtailed[111]. In the United Kingdom such restrictions have markedly reduced the incidence of amphetamine abuse and psychosis.

Chlorphentermine has been withdrawn from the market and thus need not be considered further.

Glucagon, although possibly effective, is likely to prove unacceptable in terms of side effects; this together with the need for frequent intramuscular administration would preclude its routine use in obesity.

Thus, of the drugs listed at the beginning of this chapter, only diethylpropion, phentermine, fenfluramine and mazindol remain as potentially useful anorectic agents in the treatment of obesity. Each of these will now be considered individually.

(a) Diethylpropion (Tenuate, Tepanil, Apisate)
This compound, particularly in its long acting form, is currently the anorectic drug most frequently prescribed by general practitioners in the United Kingdom[112] and in the USA[113]. It is also favoured by patients[114].

A number of double-blind controlled trials have consistently demonstrated the short-term superiority of diethylpropion to placebo in helping obese patients lose weight[21,22,115-122]. Even after five months continuous medication diethylpropion was still found to be exerting an effect[123].

Intermittent medication appears to be as effective as continuous medication[124], although a subsequent study which I undertook suggests this only holds true when the active drug is given first in the intermittent regime[125], a finding which has certain implications regarding the question of tolerance. In my study there were three regimes:

(i) Continuous diethylpropion (as Tenuate Dospan) 75 mg daily for four months.

(ii) Diethylpropion administered during the first and third months only, with placebo given during the second and fourth months.

(iii) Diethylpropion in the second and fourth months with placebo on the first and third months.

The weight loss among patients during the second months on regime (iii) was not significantly greater than that shown by those on regime (i), yet those on regime (iii) had received no active drug for the preceding month whereas the regime (i) patients had. In other words the fall in weight loss observed from the first to the second month in regime (i) was unlikely to be entirely due to pharmacological tolerance (if at all) as the same pattern of response was observed in the group in which drug tolerance could not have occurred. In addition approximately twice as much weight was lost each month by the patients on the continuous regime as by the patients who happened to be on placebo for that month (Figure 7.8).

There have been three clinical trials in which diethylpropion has been compared to fenfluramine; in two the long acting form of diethylpropion 75 mg once daily was compared with thrice daily fenfluramine 20 mg[126] or 40 mg[127]; in both of these diethylpropion appeared somewhat more effective than fenfluramine. In the third trial thrice daily diethylpropion 25 mg was used, and no differnce in weight loss was observed between the two drugs[128]. Trials such as these in which a fixed dose of one drug is compared with a fixed dose of another have certain limitations. All one can deduce from them is that a given dose of one drug is better, worse or equal to a fixed dose of the other. What is more important clinically is

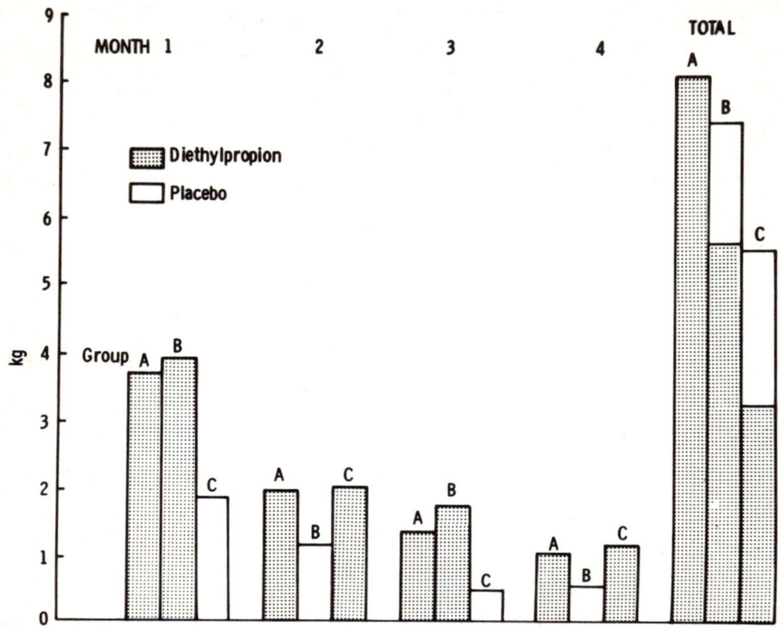

FIGURE 7.8 The pattern of weight loss in obese patients over a four-month period following continuous diethylpropion (group A—26 patients) intermittent diethylpropion, starting with active medication (group B—27 patients); intermittent diethylpropion, starting with placebo (group C—28 patients)

whether one drug is more effective than another not only in terms of weight loss but also in terms of acceptability and side effects when given in an optimum dosage; the optimum dose is likely to vary widely from patient to patient.

Although diethylpropion is not as centrally stimulating as amphetamine, it does have some central stimulant activity. The effect of diethylpropion on critical flicker fusion, a measure of central arousal, is similar to that of known stimulant compounds such as amphetamine[129,130]. Diethylpropion also has some effect on the EEG during sleep but this is less than that produced by other anorectic drugs[131]; clinically we found that an evening dose of 25 mg diethylpropion did not affect the subjective evaluation of sleep as compared with an evening placebo tablet under double blind conditions[132]. Some patients, however, do notice greater difficulty in getting off to sleep and a few remark on other central effects[123]. Other commonly reported side effects reflect the sympathomimetic action of the drug, of these dryness of the mouth is the most common.

Finally, diethylpropion has been abused, although this seems to be a rare occurrence; when it does happen an amphetamine-like psychosis may result[133-135].

In summary, diethylpropion, particularly in its long acting form in a dose of 75 mg daily, appears to be a clinically useful anorectic agent in the treatment of obesity.

(b) Phentermine (Duromine, Ionamin)

Double-blind clinical trials show a clear superiority of phentermine, given as a single daily dose of 30 mg over placebo[136-139]. Intermittent phentermine appears to be as effective as continuous administration[138,139], and it is also as effective as dexamphetamine[140] and as continuous fenfluramine 20 mg thrice daily[138].

The commonest side effect of phentermine is insomnia, presumably a reflection of its central stimulant properties.

(c) Fenfluramine (Ponderax, Ponderal, Pondomin)

Fenfluramine is a most interesting compound, for although structurally resembling amphetamine, the introduction of the CF_3 radicle markedly affects its pharmacology. We have already seen that it is a potent anorectic drug[31], with its anorectic action mediated by 5-hydroxytryptamine[74,89-92]. In contrast to amphetamine it is not a central stimulant[141]; it is if anything a depressant[142] and can itself counter the stimulant effect of amphetamine on critical flicker fusion[143]. Clinically it can precipitate overt depressive symptoms[144].

A number of well conducted double blind clinical trials have shown a clear cut superiority of fenfluramine, administered as an oral dose of 60-120 mg daily in divided doses, over placebo in helping obese patients lose weight[145-151]. Its clinical efficacy, and presumably its anorectic effect, persists for many weeks[149]. When compared with other anorectic drugs in fixed dose studies (the limitations of which have been discussed) it appears equivalent to dexamphetamine sulphate[148], superior to metformin[150] (a drug which probably has no direct anorectic action, see above), equivalent to mazindol[151] and somewhat less effective than the long-acting form of diethylpropion[126,127].

In contrast to phentermine and diethylpropion, where intermittent therapy was found to be as effective as continuous therapy, intermittent treatment with fenfluramine is not as good as continuous treatment[139]. This comparative ineffectiveness of intermittent fenfluramine is probably at least partly related to the tendency for a rebound depressive mood swing to occur on withdrawal of fenfluramine. In fact withdrawal depression has now become a well recognised potential danger in the treatment of obesity with fenfluramine[152,153] and it should therefore not be used in patients with a tendency to develop depressive symptoms[154]. Because of this tendency to produce withdrawal depression fenfluramine medication should not be stopped abruptly; a gradual tailing off in dosage is preferable.

Where fenfluramine is particularly useful is in the management of phenothiazine-induced obesity. Many psychiatric patients who are maintained on long-term treatment with phenothiazine compounds find that they eat more, and consequently gain weight, as a result of a markedly increased appetite. Studies have shown that fenfluramine can either reverse or prevent such a phenothiazine-induced weight gain[94]. This finding has considerable theoretical significance when considered in the light of the observation that other phenylethylamine derivatives do not counter phenothiazine-induced obesity. Such clinical findings are consistent with animal data suggesting a different neurochemical mode of action of fenfluramine from that of the other anorectic drugs with a phenylethylamine structure.

The metabolic action of fenfluramine on peripheral muscle tissue both *in vitro* and *in vivo*[96] has already been mentioned. At one time it was claimed that the efficacy of fenfluramine in obesity was due at least in part to this action but metabolic studies in patients have failed to confirm this[97,98]. Weight loss was the same on a given diet whether or not fenfluramine was administered, suggesting that fenfluramine acts clinically by virtue of its anorectic effect rather than by any metabolic activity it may possess.

Fenfluramine would appear to have a direct action on the gastrointestinal tract, for gastrointestinal symptoms such as nausea and diarrhoea are more common during fenfluramine treatment than with other anorectic drugs such as diethylpropion[126,127]. The pharmacological basis for this remains obscure. In order to minimise such symptoms it is recommended that the dose is gradually built up from 20 mg twice daily to a maximum of 40 mg three times daily.

Overdosage of fenfluramine has proved fatal in children[155,156]. In adults an abnormal mental state develops which differs from that seen with amphetamine or diethylpropion intoxication, in that relaxation, rather than stimulation is prominent, and visual rather than auditory hallucinations occur[157]. These symptoms have been sought after by some individuals, particularly in South Africa where fenfluramine was at one time available without prescription; following restriction of its supply the incidence of fenfluramine abuse has fallen. Apart from a short-lived flurry of abuse in the Cardiff area of Wales there has been very little tendency towards illicit consumption of fenfluramine and it is not generally recognised as a substance which is prone to lead to drug dependence or abuse.

In summary fenfluramine can be considered as an effective anorectic agent, being particularly useful in the treatment of the over-anxious and tense type of obese patient. It should, however, only be used with caution in patients with a history of depression. Fenfluramine would appear to be the drug of choice in the management of phenothiazine-induced obesity.

(d) Mazindol (Teronac, Sanorex)

Mazindol is the most recently introduced of the clinically available anorectic drugs. Its chemical structure differs from that of the other anorectic drugs we have considered in this section and it has been suggested that its mode of action also differs, although this is as yet not fully confirmed. Clinically, mazindol in a dose of 1 mg three times daily or as a single daily dose of 2 mg has been found to be superior to placebo[36,158-161], but in at least one trial the difference between mazindol 2 mg daily and placebo failed to reach significance, although the reduction in skinfold thickness was significantly greater with mazindol[163]. As with phentermine and diethylpropion intermittent therapy proved as effective as continuous[158]. Mazindol in a dose of 1 mg thrice daily appears to be at least as effective as dextroamphetamine sulphate 5 mg thrice daily[159], phenmetrazine 25 mg thrice daily[158] and fenfluramine in a dose up to 120 mg a day[151]; appetite suppression was reported as 'moderate' after both mazindol and dextroamphetamine[159]. It can produce tachycardia but has no obvious central stimulating effect as measured by critical flicker fusion[163], however subjective stimulation effects and insomnia have been reported in clinical studies[159].

Further comparative trials and direct analysis of its anorectic action are required before the place of mazindol in the management of obesity can be established.

Clinical use of anorectic drugs

(i) When to use them

Opinion regarding the value of anorectic drugs in the treatment of obesity varies widely. On the one hand are those authorities who dismiss such preparations out of hand as being at best useless, and at worst dangerous[164-166]; on the other hand there are those, equally eminent, who point to the considerable help such drugs may be to obese patients[167]. Most writers on the subject take a middle view; they consider that anorectic drugs do have a definite, if limited place, in the treatment of obesity, although even here some authors are rather more enthusiastic than others[168-171]. Whatever the pundits say, the majority of patients certainly find such drugs helpful[114], and doctors respond to this experience of their patients. In one recent survey it was found that 78% of general practitioners prescribed anorectic drugs[113].

My own view is that anorectic drugs can be used with benefit to help obese patients, but they should neither be the sole nor the initial treatment. In the first instance suitable dietary advice and, where necessary counselling along behaviourist lines (see Chapter 6) should be tried. It is only when patients cease to respond to such measures that anorectic drugs should be considered. Even then they can only be thought of as an adjunct to dietary control.

Anorectic drugs should not be used in patients with a past history of drug abuse, nor in that relatively uncommon group of patients whose eating behaviour is so bizarre as to fall into the category of the grossly pathological. Such patients are likely to develop dependence to the drug without obtaining any corresponding benefit from it in terms of weight loss; for them long-term psychiatric treatment is the only approach likely to lead to any success[165].

Although some authors have described the value of anorectic drugs in severe childhood obesity[172], others have found such preparations to have little value in children[9]. Furthermore there have been disturbing reports suggesting that administration of appetite suppressant drugs to children can lead to stunting of growth[173,174]. In the light of these findings I consider it inadvisable to prescribe these drugs for anyone under the age of sixteen.

(*ii*) *Which drug to use*

Of the four available compounds which we considered as having potential value (diethylpropion, phentermine, fenfluramine and mazindol), the relative place of mazindol must remain uncertain until direct assessment of its anorectic effect has been undertaken and more extensive comparative clinical studies have been completed.

If there is evidence of depressive symptoms present, or a past history of a depressive episode then fenfluramine is contra-indicated. For such patients diethylpropion in the long-acting form 75 mg daily or phentermine 15-30 mg daily are the anorectic drugs of choice. Both are as effective when given intermittently as when given continuously and, on the grounds that tolerance and dependence are less likely to occur, intermittent medication is preferable to continuous. Periods of four to six weeks on active treatment with intervening drug-free periods of two to four weeks should prove suitable for the majority of patients for whom, in the light of the considerations discussed above, it has been decided to prescribe an anorectic drug.

Fenfluramine, 20-40 mg three times daily or 60-120 mg daily as the long acting form, is particularly useful in the over-active, tense obese patient in whom the mild stimulant activity of diethylpropion and phentermine may prove distressing. Fenfluramine has also been said to be particularly useful in obese diabetics[175]. In addition it is probably the most effective drug in the management of phenothiazine-induced obesity (see above).

Fenfluramine, in contrast to diethylpropion and phentermine, should not be administered intermittently because of the increased risk of precipitating withdrawal depression.

CONCLUSIONS

The ideal anorectic drug, which guarantees long-term continuous reduction of calorie intake without any risk of side-effects, tolerance or drug dependence, has yet to be discovered. In any case this is by no means the only possible pharmacological approach to the problem of obesity. Drugs which increase calorie expenditure (thermogenic drugs) might prove to be more useful. Unfortunately those that have been tried in the past have tended to be too toxic. Recent work, however, has indicated that there may be a very small proportion of obese patients whose resting metabolic rate is so low that they can benefit from judicious administration of a thyroid hormone[176]. Other thermogenic drugs are continuously being sought and one eventually may be found which harmlessly and effortlessly raises energy expenditure.

Whatever the future holds, in the present state of knowledge I am of the opinion that anorectic drugs can play a useful part in the overall management of obesity, but they should never be regarded as the only treatment. After all an anorectic drug is basically a pharmacological device designed to help obese patients keep to their reducing diets more easily by reducing their desire for food. Patients should always be given the opportunity to see how well they can maintain a dietary regime without pharmacological assistance before drug treatment is considered.

All of the truly anorectic drugs considered in this review have been shown to produce effects on the central nervous system over and above their anorectic action, with the majority causing stimulation. In fact, at one time, it was suggested that, if anorectic drugs were effective in obesity, it was entirely by virtue of their central stimulant properties[177]. We now know that this is not the case; at least one potent anorectic compound, fenfluramine, has no stimulant properties whatsoever, it is, if anything, a depressant.

Further study of the interaction between the anorectic properties of a drug and its mood elevating or lowering properties could well throw light on the neurophysiological mechanisms underlying both affect and hunger. Pursuit of these problems, using the techniques of both clinical and experimental pharmacology is, in my opinion, likely to prove a most valuable approach. It is only by asking human subjects how they feel that we can gain any insight into the subjective changes produced by a drug, and it is only by examining the neurochemical and neurophysiological changes produced by the same drug in the central nervous system of experimental animals that we can gain any idea of how it works. Feeding behaviour is particularly amenable to such a dual approach, and research along such lines may well provide the answer to the long-standing question, 'Why do we eat?' Only when we have the answer to that, shall we be in a position to implement a truly rational pharmacological treatment for obesity.

REFERENCES

1. Alles, G. A. (1927). Comparative physiological action of phenylethanolamine. *J. Pharmacol.,* **32,** 121
2. Printzmetal, M. and Bloomberg, W. (1935). The use of benzedrine for the treatment of narcolepsy. *J. Amer. Med. Ass.,* **105,** 2051
3. Ulrich, H. (1937). Narcolepsy and its treatment with benzedrine sulphate. *New Eng. J. Med.,* **217,** 696
4. Nathanson, M. H. (1937). The central action of beta-aminopropylbenzene (benzedrine). *J. Amer. Med. Ass.,* **108,** 528
5. Davidoff, E. and Reifenstein, E. C. (1937). The stimulating action of benzedrine sulphate. *J. Amer. Med. Ass.,* **108,** 1770
6. Lesses, M. F. and Myerson, A. (1938). Benzedrine sulphate as an aid to the treatment of obesity. *New Eng. J. Med.,* **218,** 119
7. Ivy, A. C. and Krasno, L. R. (1941). Amphetamine sulphate: a review of the pharmacology. *War Med.,* **1,** 15
8. Silverstone, J. T. (1967). The measurement of hunger in relation to food intake. Proceedings VII International Cong. Nutrition, Hamburg
9. Bruch, H. and Waters, I. (1942). Benzedrine sulphate (amphetamine) in the treatment of obese children and adolescents. *J. Pediat.,* **20,** 54
10. Bahnsen, P., Jacobsen, E. and Thesleff, H. (1938). The subjective effect of beta-phenylisopropylaminsulphate on normal adults. *Acta Med. Scand.,* **97,** 89
11. Jacobsen, E. and Wollstein, A. (1939). Studies on the subjective

effects of the cephalotropic amines in men. *Acta Med. Scand.*, **100,** 159

12. Harris, S. C., Ivy, A. C. and Searle, L. M. (1947). The mechanism of amphetamine-induced loss of weight. *J. Amer. Med. Ass.,* **134,** 1468
13. Bernstein, L. M. and Grossman, M. I. (1956). An experimental test of the glucostatic theory of regulation of food intake. *J. Clin. Invest.,* **35,** 627
14. Silverstone, J. T. and Stunkard, A. J. (1968). The anorectic effect of dexamphetamine sulphate. *Brit. J. Pharmacol. Chemother.,* **33,** 513
15. Fineberg, S. K. (1959). Obesity and diabetes: a re-evaluation. *Annal. Int. Med.,* **52,** 750
16. Penick, S. B. and Hinkle, L. E. (1964). The effect of expectation in response to phenmetrazine. *Psychosomatic Med.,* **26,** 369
17. Patel, N., Mock, D. C. and Hagens, J. (1963). Comparison of benzphetamine, phenmetrazine, D-amphetamine and placebo. *Clin. Pharmacol. Ther.,* **4,** 330
18. Freed, S. C., Hays, E. E. (1959). A new non-amphetamine anorectic agent. *Amer. J. Med. Sci.,* 55
19. Seaton, D. A., Rose, K. and Duncan L. J. P. (1964). A comparison of the appetite suppressing properties of D-amphetamine and phentermine. *Scot. Med. J.,* **9,** 482
20. Silverstone, J. T. (1972). The anorectic effect of a long-acting preparation of phentermine (Duromine). *Psychopharmacologia,* **25,** 315
21. Haden, D. R. and Lucy, C. (1961). Diethylpropion in the treatment of obesity: a crossover trial of a long-acting preparation. *Ulster Med. J.,* **30,** 109
22. Cunningham, G. L. W. (1963). Diethylpropion in the treatment of obesity. *J. Coll. Gen. Pract.,* **6,** 347
23. Silverstone, J. T. (1968). The evaluation of appetite suppressant drugs. Third International Conference on the Regulation of Food and Water Intake
24. Silverstone, J. T., Turner, P. and Humpherson, P. (1968). Direct measurement of the anorectic activity of diethylpropion (Tenuate Dospan). *J. Clin. Pharmacol.,* **8,** 172
25. Fineberg, S. K. (1962). Evaluation of anorexigenic agents. *Amer. J. Clin. Nutr.,* **11,** 509
26. Jackson, I. M. D. and Whyte, W. O. (1965). Chlorphentermine-SA in the treatment of obesity and the effect of weight loss on steroid excretion. *Brit. Med. J.,* **ii,** 453

27. Le Douarec, J.-C. and Schmitt, H. (1964). Pharmacological comparison of seven anorectic drugs. *Therapie,* **19,** 831
28. Duncan, E. H., Hyde, C. A., Regan, N. A. and Sweetman,B. (1965). A preliminary trial of fenfluramine in general practice. *Brit. J. Clin. Pract.,* **19,** 451
29. Munro, J. F., Seaton, D. A. and Duncan, L. J. P. (1966). Treatment of refractory obesity with fenfluramine. *Brit. Med. J.,* **ii,** 624
30. Sainani, G. S. and Fulambarkar, A. M. (1973). A double-blind clinical trial of fenfluramine in the treatment of obesity. *Brit. J. Clin. Pract.,* **27,** 136
31. Silverstone, J. T., Fincham, J. and Campbell, D. B. (1974). The anorectic activity of fenfluramine. *Postgrad. Med. J.* (*Supplement*) (In press)
32. Campbell, D. B. (1972). Absorption, distribution and metabolism of fenfluramine. *Vie Med. Canad.,* **19**
33. Holmstrand, J. (1974). Subjective effects of the anorexogenic agents—fenfluramine and AN 448—in normal subjects. *Postgrad. Med. J.* (*Supplement*) (In press)
34. De Felice, E. a., Bronstein, S. and Cohen, A. (1969). Double-blind comparison of placebo and 42-548, a new appetite suppressant in obese volunteers. *Cur. Ther. Res.,* **11,** 256
35. Kornhaber, A. (1973). Obesity-depression: clinical evaluation with a new anorexigenic agent. *Psychosomatics,* **14,** 162
36. Grapin, B. and Cohen, A. (1974). Drug therapy in simple obesity: controlled trial of mazindol. *Internat. Med. Digest,* **9,** 15
37. Simeons, A. J. W. (1954). The action of chorionic gonadotrophin in the obese. *Lancet,* **i,** 946
38. Carne, S. (1961). The action of chorionic gonadotrophin in the obese. *Lancet,* **ii,** 1282
39. Frank, B. W. (1964). The use of chorionic gonadotrophin hormone in the treatment of obesity. *Amer. J. Clin. Nut.,* **14,** 133
40. Asher, W. L. and Harper, H. W. (1973). Effect of human chorionic gonadotrophin on weight loss, hunger and feeling of well-being. *Amer. J. Clin. Nutr.,* **26,** 211
41. Hirsch, J. and Van Itallie, T. B. (1973). The treatment of obesity. *Amer. J. Clin. Nutr.,* **26,** 1039
42. Roginsky, M. S. and Barnett, J. (1966). Double-blind study of phenethyldiguanide (phenformin) on weight control of obese non-diabetic subjects. *Amer. J. Clin. Nutr.,* **19,** 223

43. Hart, A. and Cohen, H. (1970). Treatment of obese non-diabetic patients with phenformin. A double-blind cross-over trial. *Brit. Med. J.,* **i,** 22
44. Munro, J. F., MacCuish, A. C., Marshall, A., Wilson, E. and Duncan, L. J. P. (1969). Weight-reducing effect of diguanides in obese non-diabetic women. *Lancet,* **ii,** 13
45. Penick, S. B. and Hinkle, L. (1963). The effect of glucagon, phenmetrazine and epinephrine on hunger, food intake and plasma NEFA. *Amer. J. Clin. Nutr.,* **13,** 110
46. Penick, S. B., Smith, G. P., Wieneke, K. and Hinkle, L. E. (1963). Experimental evaluation between hunger and gastric motility. *Amer. J. Physiol.,* **205**
47. Duncan, L. J. P., Rose, K. and Meiklejohn, A. P. (1960). Phenmetrazine HCL and methyl cellulose in the treatment of 'refractory' obesity. *Lancet,* **i,** 1262
48. Hossain, M., Campbell, D. B. (1974). Fenfluramine and methyl cellulose in the treatment of obesity. *Postgrad. Med. J.* (*Supplement*) (In press)
49. Anand, B. K. (1961). Nervous regulation of food intake. *Physiol. Rev.,* **41,** 677
50. Albert, D. J., Storlein, L. H. (1969). Hyperphagia in rats with cuts between the ventromedial and lateral hypothalamus. *Science,* **165,** 599
51. Morgane, P. J. (1961). Medial forebrain bundle and 'feeding centres' of the hypothalamus. *J. Comp. Neurol.,* **117,** 1
52. Morgane, P. J. and Jacobs, H. L. (1969). Hunger and satiety. *World Review of Nutrition and Dietetics,* **1,** 100
53. Ungerstedt, U. (1971). Adipsia and aphagia after 6-hydroxydopamine-induced degeneration of the nigro-striatal dopamine system. *Acta Physiol. Scand. Suppl.,* **367,** 95
54. Gold, R. M. (1973). Hypothalamic obesity: the myth of the ventromedial nucleus. *Science,* **182,** 488
55. Ungerstedt, U. (1971). Stereotaxic mapping of the monoamine pathways in the rat brain. *Acta Physiol. Scan. Suppl.,* **367,** 1
56. Morgane, P. J. (1968). The function of the limbic forebrain-limbic midbrain system in the regulation of food and water intake. *Ann. N. Y. Acad. Sci.,* **157,** 806
57. Grossman, S. P. and Grossman, L. (1973). Persisting deficits in rats 'recovered' from transections of fibres which enter or leave hypothalamus laterally. *J. Comp. Physiol. Psychol.,* **85,** 515

58. Hervey, G. R. (1971). Physiological mechanisms for the regulation of energy balance. *Proc. Nutr. Soc.,* **30,** 109
59. LeMagnen, J., Devos, M., Gaudilliere, J.-P., Louis-Sylvestre, J. and Tallon, S. (1973). Role of a lipostatic mechanism in regulation by feeding of energy balance in rats. *J. Comp. Physiol. Psychol.,* **84,** 1
60. Grossman, S. P. (1969). A neuropharmacological analysis of hypothalamic and extra-hypothalamic mechanisms concerned with the regulation of food and water intake. *Ann. N.Y. Acad. Sci.,* **157,** 902
61. Booth, D. A. (1968). Mechanism of action of norepinephrine in eliciting an eating response on injections into the rat hypothalamus. *J. Pharmacol. Exp. Ther.,* **160,** 336
62. Ahlskog, J. E., Hoebel, B. G. (1973). Overeating and obesity from damage to a noradrenergic system in the brain. *Science,* **182,** 166
63. Leibowitz, S. F. (1970). Reciprocal hunger-regulating circuits involving alpha and beta-adrenergic receptors located, respectively, in the ventromedial and lateral hypothalamus. *Proc. Nat. Acad. Sci. Wash.,* **67,** 1063
64. Baile, C. A. and Forbes, J. M. (1974). Control of feed intake and regulation of energy balance in ruminants. *Physiol. Rev.,* **54,** 160
65. Hoebel, B. G. (1971). Feeding: neural control of intake. *Ann. Rev. Psychol.,* **33,** 533
66. Goldman, W. and Lehr, D. (1971). Suppression of eating and enhancement of drinking induced by Serotonin (5HT) and abolition of these effects by b-adrenergic blockade. *Fed. Proc.,* **30,** 503
67. Fitzsimons, J. T. (1972). Thirst. *Physiol. Rev.,* **52,** 468
68. Mawson, A. R. (1974). Anorexia nervosa and the regulation of intake: a review. *Psychol. Med.,* **4,** 289
69. Printzmetal, M. and Alles, G. A. (1940). The central nervous system stimulant effects of dextro-amphetamine sulphate. *Amer. J. Med. Sci.,* **200,** 665
70. Baez, L. A. (1974). Role of catecholamines in the anorectic effects of amphetamine in rats. *Psychopharmacologia,* **35,** 91
71. Fibiger, H. C., Zis, A. P. and McGeer, E. G. (1973). Feeding and drinking deficits after 6-hydroxydopamine administration in the rat: similarities to the lateral hypothalamic syndrome. *Brain Res.,* **55,** 135
72. Zigmond, M. J. and Stricker, E. M. (1973). Recovery of feeding

and drinking by rats afer intraventricular 6-hydroxydopamine in lateral hypothalamic lesions. *Science,* **182,** 717

73. Barzaghi, F., Gropetti, A., Mantegazza, P. and Muller, E. E. (1973). Reduction of food intake by apomorphine: a pimozide-sensitive effect. *J. Pharm. Pharmacol.,* **25,** 909

74. Kruk, Z. L. (1973). Dopamine and 5-hydroxytryptamine inhibit feeding in rats. *Nature* (*New Biol.*), **246,** 52

75. Bunney, B. S., Aghajanian, G. K. and Roth, R. H. (1973). Comparison of effects of l-dopa, amphetamine and apomorphine on firing rate of rat dopaminergic neurones. *Nature* (*New Biol.*), **245,** 123

76. Carlsson, A. (1970). Amphetamine and brain catecholamines in *Amphetamines and Related Compounds,* p. 289 (E. Costa and S. Garattini, editors) (New York: Raven)

77. Cole, S. D. (1973). Hypothalamic feeding mechanisms and amphetamine anorexia. *Psychol. Bull.,* **79,** 13

78. Epstein, A. (1970). Suppression of eating and drinking by amphetamine and other drugs in normal and hyperphagic rats. *J. Comp. Physiol. Psychol.,* **72,** 60

79. Carlisle, H. J. (1964). Differential effects of amphetamine on food and water intake in rats with lateral hypothalamic lesions. *J. Comp. Physiol.,* **58,** 47

80. Reid, A. A. (1964). Pharmacological antagonism between chlorpromazine and phenmetrazine in mental hospital patients. *Med. J. Aust.,* **i,** 187

81. Sletten, I. W., Ognjanov, V., Menendez, S., Sundland, D. and El-Toumi, A. (1967). Weight reduction with chlorphentermine and phenmetrazine in obese psychiatric patients during chlorpromazine therapy. *Curr. Ther. Res.,* **9,** 570

82. Becker, B. A. (1959). Pharmacological activity of phenyl-tert.-butylamine. *Fed. Proc.,* **18,** 1448

83. Yelnosky, J., Panasevich, R. E., Borrelli, A. R. and Lawlor, R. B. (1969). Pharmacology of phentermine. *Arch. Int. Pharmacodyn.,* **178,** 62

84. Stark, P. and Totty, C. W. (1967). Effects of amphetamine on eating elicited by hypothalamic stimulation. *J. Pharmacol. Exp. Therap.,* **158,** 272

85. Cullen, P. D. and Swartz, H. A. (1964). Anorectic agents: the effect on food intake, oxygen consumption and weight loss in gold thioglucose-obese and normal non-obese mice. *Canad. Pharmacol. J.,* **97,** 33

86. Holm. T., Huss, I., Kopk, R., Møller Nielsen, I. and Petersen,

P. V. (1960). Pharmacology of a series of nuclear substituted phenyl-tertiary-butylamines with particular reference to anorexigenic and central stimulating properties. *Acta Pharmacol. Toxicol.,* **17,** 121

87. Møller Nielsen, I., Dubnick, B. (1970). Pharmacology of chlorphentermine in *Amphetamines and Related Compounds,* p. 63 (E. Costa and S. Garattini, editors) (New York: Raven Press)
88. Blundell, J. E. and Leshem, M. B. (1974). Hypothalamic lesions and drug-induced anorexia. *Postgraduate Med. J.* (*Supplement*) (In press)
89. Samanin, R., Ghezzi, D., Valzelli, L. and Garattini, S. (1972). The effects of selective lesioning of brain serotonin or catecholamine-containing neurones on the anorectic activity of fenfluramine and amphetamine. *Europ. J. Pharmacol.,* **19,** 318
90. Jesperson, S. and Scheel-Kruger, J. (1970). Antagonism by methysergide of the 5-hydroxytryptamine-like action of toxic doses of fenfluramine on dogs. *J. Pharm. Pharmacol.,* **22,** 637
91. Southgate, P. J., Mayer, S. R., Boxall, E. and Wilson, A. B. (1971). Some 5-hydroxytryptamine-like actions of fenfluramine: a comparison with (+) amphetamine and diethylpropion. *J. Pharm. Pharmacol.,* **23,** 600
92. Fuxe, K. (1974). On the *in vivo* and *in vitro* action of fenfluramine and its derivatives on central monoamine neurones, especially 5HT nerves and their relation to the anorectic activity of fenfluramine. *Postgrad. Med. J.* (*Supplement*) (In press)
93. Ghezzi, D., Ramanin, R., Bernasconi, S., Tognoni, G., Gerna, M. and Garattini, S. (1973). Effect of thymoleptics on fenfluramine-induced depletion of brain serotonin in rats. *Europ. J. Pharmacol.,* **24,** 205
94. Jensen, P. S. and Kirk, L. (1972). Fenfluramine (Ponderal) in the treatment of adipositas caused by neuroleptics. Paper presented at the Annual Meeting of the Scandinavian Society of Psychopharmacology, Copenhagen
95. Kirby, M. J. and Turner, P. (1974). Fenfluramine and norfenfluramine on glucose uptake into skeletal muscle. *Postgrad. Med. J.* (*Supplement*) (In press)
96. Butterfield, W. J. H. and Whichelow, M. J. (1968). Fenfluramine and muscle glucose uptake in man. *Lancet,* **ii,** 109
97. Garrow, J. S., Belton, E. A. and Daniels, A. (1972). A controlled investigation of the 'glycolyptic' action of fenfluramine. *Lancet,* **ii,** 559

98. Petrie, J. C., Mowat, J. A. Bewsher, P. D. and Stowers, J. M. (1974). Metabolic effects of fenfluramine. *Postgrad. Med. J.* (*Supplement*) (In press)

99. Bizzi, A., Veneroni, E. and Garattini, S. (1973). Effect of fenfluramine on the intestinal absorption of triglycerides. *Europ. J. Pharmac.,* **23,** 131

100. Sandoz Pharmaceuticals. (1973). 'Sanorex' (Mazindol): a new anorexiant. Product Monograph

101. Smart, J. V. and Turner, P. (1966). Influence of urinary pH on the degree and duration of action of amphetamine on the critical flicker fusion frequency in man. *Brit. J. Pharmacol. Chemotherap.,* **26,** 468

102. Besser, G. N. (1967). Auditory flutter fusion as a measure of the actions of centrally acting drugs: modification of the threshold for fusion and the influence of adapting stimuli. *Brit. J. Pharmacol. Chemotherap.,* **30,** 329

103. Connell, P. H. (1966). Clinical manifestations and treatment of amphetamine type of dependence. *J. Amer. Med. Ass.,* **196,** 130

104. Evans, J. (1959). Psychosis and addiction to phenmetrazine (Preludin). *Lancet,* **ii,** 152

105. Connell, P. H. (1958). Amphetamine Psychosis. *Maudsley Monographs,* **5,** London

106. Bell, D. S. (1965). Comparison of amphetamine psychosis and schizophrenia. *Brit. J. Psychiat.,* **111,** 701

107. Jonsson, L. E. and Gunne, L.-M. (1970). Clinical studies of amphetamine psychosis in *Amphetamine and Related Compounds,* p. 929 (E. Costa and S. Garattini, editors) (New York: Raven Press)

108. Griffith, J. D., Cavanaugh, J., Held, J. and Oates, J. A. (1972). Dextroamphetamine: evaluation of psychomimetic properties in man. *Arch. Gen Psychiat.,* **26,** 97

109. Angrist, B. M., Shopsin, B. and Gershon, S. (1971). Comparative psychotomimetic effects of stereoisomers of amphetamine. *Nature,* **234,** 152

110. Anderson, J. (1974). Drugs and appetite. *Practitioner,* **212,** 536

111. British Medical Journal. (1968). Control of amphetamine preparations. *Brit. Med. J.,* **iv,** 572

112. Craddock, D. (1973). *Obesity and its Management* (2nd edition) (Edinburch: Churchill Livingstone)

113. Lasagna, L. (1973). Attitudes towards appetite suppressants: a survey of U.S. physicians. *J. Amer. Med. Ass.,* **225,** 44

114. Ashwell, M. A. (1973). A survey of patients' views on doctors' treatment of obesity. *Practitioner,* **211,** 653
115. Decina, L., Tanyol, H. (1960). Treatment of obesity with a new anorexiant, diethylpropion, without special stress on diet. *N.Y. State J. Med.,* **60,** 2702
116. Rosenberg, B. A. (1961). A double-blind study of diethylpropion in obesity. *Am. J. Med. Sci.,* **242,** 201
117. Seaton, D. A., Duncan, L. J. P., Rose, K. and Scott, A. M. (1961). Diethylpropion in the treatment of 'refractory obesity'. *Brit. Med. J.,* **i,** 1009
118. de Ramos, E. C. (1964). The use of diethylpropion in the treatment of obesity. *Brit. J. Clin. Pract.,* **18**
119. Russek, H. I. (1966). Control of obesity in patients with angina pectoris; a double-blind study with diethylpropion hydrochloride. *Amer. J. Med. Sci.,* **251,** 461
120. Williams, J. (1968). Trial of a long-acting preparation of diethylpropion in obese diabetics. *Practitioner,* **200,** 411
121. Noble, R. E. (1971). A controlled study of a weight reduction regimen. *Curr. Ther. Res.,* **13,** 685
122. Bolding, O. T. (1974). Diethylpropion hydrochloride; an effective appetite suppressant. *Curr. Ther. Res.,* **16,** 40
123. McKay, R. H. G. (1973). Long-term use of diethylpropion in obesity. *Curr. Med. Res.,* **1,** 489
124. Le Riche, W. H. and Csima, A. (1967). A long-acting appetite suppressant drug. *Canad. Med. Ass. J.,* **97,** 1016
125. Silverstone, J. T. (1974). Intermittent treatment with anorectic drugs. *Practitioner,* **212,** 245
126. Silverstone, J. T., Cooper, R. M., and Begg, R. R. (1970). A comparative trial of fenfluramine and diethylpropion in obesity. *Brit. J. Clin. Pract.,* **24,** 423
127. Van Rooyen, R. J. and Van Der Merwe, M. (1971). Comparison of diethylpropion (Tenuate Dospan) and fenfluramine. *Med. Proc.,* **17,** 420
128. Follows, O. J. (1971). A comparative trial of fenfluramine and diethylpropion in obese, hypertensive patients. *Brit. J. Clin. Pract.,* **25,** 236
129. Smart, J. V., Sneddon, J. M. and Turner, P. (1967). A comparison of the effects of chlorphentermine, diethylpropion and phenmetrazine on critical flicker frequency. *Brit. J. Pharmacol. Chemother.,* **30,** 307
130. Sjoberg, L. and Jonsson, C.-O. (1967). Studies in the

psychological effects of a new drug (diethylpropion). *Scan J. Psychol.,* **8,** 81

131. Lewis, S. A. (1970). Comparative effects of some amphetamine derivatives on human sleep in *Amphetamines and Related Compounds,* p. 873 (E. Costa and S. Garattini, editors) (New York: Raven Press)
132. Silverstone, J. T. and Cleary, T. (1967). A controlled trial of an evening dose of diethylpropion (Tenuate) in the treatment of obesity. *Clin. Trials J.,* **4,** 837
133. Clein, L. and Benady, D. R. (1962). Case of diethylpropion addiction. *Brit. Med. J.,* **ii,** 456
134. Jones, H. S. (1968). Diethylpropion dependence. *Med. J. Aust.,* **i,** 267
135. Whitlock, F. A. and Nadorfi, M. I. (1970). Diethylpropion and psychosis. *Med. J. Aust.,* **ii,** 1097
136. Sproule, B. C. (1969). Double blind trial of anorectic agents. *Med. J. Aust.,* **i,** 394
137. Munro, J. F., MacCuish, A. C., Wilson, E. M., and Duncan, L. J. P. (1968). Comparison of continuous and intermittent therapy in obesity. *Brit. Med. J.,* **i,** 352
138. Truant, A. P., Olon, L. P., Cobb, S. (1972). Phentermine resin as an adjunct in medical weight reduction: a controlled randomized double-blind prospective study. *Curr. Ther. Res.,* **14,** 726
139. Steel, J. M., Munro, J. F. and Duncan, L. J. P. (1973). A comparative trial of different regimens of fenfluramine and phentermine in obesity. *Practitioner,* **211,** 232
140. Le Riche, H. (1960). A study of appetite suppressants in a general practice. *Canad. Med. Ass. J.,* **82,** 467
141. Hill, R. C. and Turner, P. (1967). Fenfluramine and critical flicker frequency. *J. Pharm. Pharmacol.,* **19,** 337
142. Reuter, C. J. (1974). A review of the CNS effects of fenfluramine, 780 SE and nor-fenfluramine on animals and man. *Postgrad. Med. J.* (*Supplement*) (*In press*)
143. Turner, P. (1971). Further studies on the human pharmacology of fenfluramine. *S. Af. Med. J.,* **45,** Suppl. 13, 13
144. Imlah, N. (1970). Unusual effect of fenfluramine. *Brit. Med. J.,* **ii,** 178
145. Brodbin, P. and O'Connor, C. A. (1967). A double-blind trial of an appetite depressant, fenfluramine, in general practice. *Practitioner,* **198,** 707
146. Hollingsworth, D. R. and Amatruda, T. T. (1969). Toxic and

therapeutic effects of EMTP (fenfluramine) in obesity. *J. Clin. Pharmacol. Therap.*, **10**, 540
147. Hungerford, R. L. (1974). A comparative study of obesity in the Maori and non Maori using fenfluramine. *Postgrad. Med. J.* (*Supplement*) (In press)
148. Stunkard, A., Rickels, K. and Hesbacher, P. (1973). Fenfluramine in the treatment of obesity. *Lancet,* **i,** 503
149. Munro, J. F., MacCuish, A. G., Marshall, A., Wilson, E. M. and Duncan, L. J. P. (1966). Fenfluramine in the treatment of refractory obesity. *Brit. Med. J.,* **ii,** 624
150. Lawson, A. A. H., Roscoe, P., Strong, J. A., Gibson, A. and Petrie, P. (1970). Comparison of fenfluramine and metformin in the treatment of obesity. *Lancet,* **ii,** 437
151. Goldrick, R. B., Nester, P. J. and Havenstein, N. (1974). Comparison of a new anorectic agent AN 448 with fenfluramine in the treatment of refractory obesity. *Med. J. Aust.,* **i,** 882
152. Steel, J. M. and Briggs, M. (1972). Withdrawal depression in obese patients after fenfluramine treatment. *Brit. Med. J.,* **iii,** 26
153. Harding, T. (1972). Depression following fenfluramine withdrawal. *Brit. J. Psychiat.,* **121,** 338
154. Gaind, R. (1969). Fenfluramine (Ponderax) in the treatment of obese psychiatric outpatients. *Brit. J. Psychiat.,* **115,** 963
155. Gold, R. G., Gordon, H. E., da Costa, R. W. D., Porters, I. B. and Kimber, K. J. (1969). Fenfluramine overdosage. *Lancet,* **ii,** 1306
156. Fleisher, M. R. and Campbell, D. B. (1969). Fenfluramine overdosage. *Lancet,* **ii,** 1306
157. Levin, A. (1974). The non-medical abuse of fenfluramine by drug dependent young South Africans. *Postgrad. Med. J.* (*Supplement*) (In press)
158. Conte, A. (1973). Evaluation of Sanorex—a new appetite suppressant. *Obesity and Bariatric Medicine,* **2,** 104
159. De Felice, E. A., Chaykin, L. B., Cohen, A. (1973). Double-blind clinical evaluation of mazindol, dextroamphetamine and placebo in treatment of exogenous obesity. *Curr. Ther. Res.,* **15,** 358
160. Sharma, R. K., Collip, P. J., Rezvani, I., Strimas, J., Maddaiah, V. T. and Rezvani, E. (1973). Clinical evaluation of the anorexic activity and safety of 42-548 in children. *Clin. Paediat.,* **12,** 145
161. Smith, D. E. (1974). A new anorexiant. *Rocky Mt. Med. J.,* 41

162. Hadler, A. J. (1972). Mazindol, a new non-amphetamine anorexigenic agent. *J. Clin. Pharmacol.,* 453
163. Hedges, A. (1972). AN 448 on critical flicker frequency and heart rate in man. *S. Afr. Med. J.,* **139**
164. Drug and Therapeutics Bulletin. (1969). The management of obesity. *Drug Therpa. Bull.,* **7,** 93
165. Bruch, H. (1974). *Obesity, Anorexia Nervosa and the Person Within.* (London: Routledge and Kegan Paul)
166. Fulton, W. W. (1969). The clinical use and abuse of amphetamines and related drugs. *Prescribers J.,* **9,** 50
167. Mayer, J. (1968). *Overweight* (New Jersey: Prentice Hall)
168. Silverstone, J. T. (1967). The treatment of obesity. *Hosp. Med.,* **1,** 594
169. Anderson, J. (1972). Obesity. *Brit. Med. J.,* **i,** 560
170. Munro, J. (1973). The management of obesity. *Brit. J. Hosp. Med.,* **10,** 8
171. Garrow, J. S. (1973). Anti-obesity drugs. *Prescribers J.,* **13,** 50
172. Corber, J. (1966). Obesity in childhood: a controlled trial of anorectic drugs. *Arch. Dis. Child.,* **41,** 309
173. Nutrition Reviews. (1973). The growth of children given stimulant drugs. *Nutrit. Rev.,* **31,** 91
174. Rayner, P. H. W. and Court, J. M. (1974). The effect of dietary restriction and anorectic drugs on linear growth velocity in childhood obesity. *Postgrad. Med. J.* (*Supplement*) (In press)
175. Samuel, P. and Burland, W. (1974). Medicinal treatment of obesity. In *Obesity* (P. Samuel, W. Burland and J. Yudkin, editors) (Edinburgh: Churchill Livingstone)
176. Garrow, J. S. (1974). *Energy Balance and Obesity in Man.* (Amsterdam: North Holland)
177. Modell, W. (1960). Status and prospect of drugs for overeating. *J. Amer. Med. Ass.,* **173,** 1131

Index